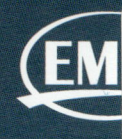

Nerve Blocks and Procedural Pain Management Guide

Editors-in-Chief
Mark F. Brady, MD, MPH | The Warren Alpert Medical School of Brown University
Donald E. Stader III, MD | Carepoint Health

Senior Editors
Andrew J. Goldsmith, MD, MBA | Brigham and Women's Hospital and Harvard Medical School
Marc L. Martel, MD | Hennepin Healthcare and University of Minnesota Medical School
Arun D. Nagdev, MD | Highland Hospital, University of California
Leland K. Perice, MD | The Warren Alpert Medical School of Brown University
Robert F. Reardon, MD | Hennepin Healthcare and University of Minnesota Medical School

Illustrator
Elena Kakoshina | www.behance.net/ArtKakos

Assistant Editors
Jenee E. Anekwe | Brown University
Jordan Brown, MD | Einstein Medical Center Philadelphia
James Tanch, MD | The Warren Alpert Medical School of Brown University

Contributors
Brendan M. Holmes, MD | The Warren Alpert Medical School of Brown University
John Martindale, MD | The Warren Alpert Medical School of Brown University
William C. Miller, MD | University of Minnesota Medical School
John Spartz, MD, MPH | Denver Health
Jeff Cords | Cords Photography
Rachel Donihoo

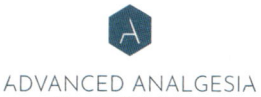

2022 EMRA Board of Directors

President Jessica Adkins Murphy, MD
President-Elect Blake Denley, MD
Immediate Past President Angela Cai, MD, MBA
Secretary/Editor, *EM Resident* Thuy Nguyen, MD
Speaker of the Council Amanda Irish, MD, MPH
Vice Speaker of the Council Michaela Banks, MD
Resident Representative to ACEP Aaron R. Kuzel, DO, MBA
Director of Education Erin Karl, MD, MEHP
Director of Health Policy Kenneth Kim, MD
Director of Leadership Development Derek Martinez, DO
Member at Large Kimberly Herard, MD
EMRA Representative to the AMA Angela Wu, MD, MPH
Medical Student Council Chair Revelle Gappy

EMRA Executive Director Kris Williams, CAE
Managing Editor Valerie Hunt

Disclaimer

This handbook is intended as a general guide to therapy only. While the editors have taken reasonable measures to ensure the accuracy of drug and dosing information presented herein, the user should consult other resources when necessary to confirm appropriate therapy, side effects, interactions, and contraindications. The publisher, authors, editors, and sponsoring organizations specifically disclaim any liability for omissions or errors found in this handbook, for appropriate use, or treatment errors. Further, although the publisher, authors, editors, and sponsoring organizations have endeavored to make this handbook comprehensive, the vast differences in emergency practice settings may necessitate treatment approaches other than those presented here.

Copyright 2023 Emergency Medicine Residents' Association
ISBN 978-1-929854-73-8
4950 W. Royal Lane, Irving, TX 75063
972.550.0920 | **emra.org**

All rights reserved. This book is protected by copyright. No part of this book may be reproduced in any form or by any means without written permission from the copyright owner.

PREFACE

The mission of Advanced Analgesia in the Emergency Department (AAED) is to provide patients with better, safer, definitive pain control. AAED is both a philosophy and an approach to pain management, integrating the best evidence-based practices into an easily understood and applicable framework emphasizing optimal patient care.

AAED appreciates the complexity and diversity of the pain experience and arms clinicians with the expertise needed to approach and ameliorate pain in all its forms. Our philosophy emphasizes these principles:
- Use of nonopioid approaches, both medications and procedures, as first-line therapies.
- An integrated approach to multimodal pain control rather than relying on monotherapies.
- Focus on realistic, functional pain management goals with patients.
- Use of empathic language and psychological interventions to improve your patients' pain experience.

AAED is based on three pillars upon which optimal pain control is provided. Once mastered, these interconnected skills and knowledge allow clinicians to be less dependent on opioid analgesics while providing patients, even those with complex injuries or co-morbidities, with optimal analgesia.

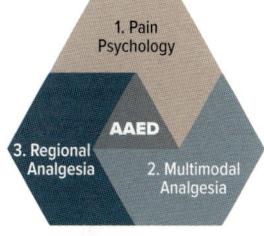

The importance of decreasing opioid utilization, especially in the context of our current opioid crisis, cannot be overstated. In this book, the regional analgesia (RA) pillar of advanced analgesia will be described and explored. We aim to help emergency clinicians build on their foundational knowledge by providing a quick, accessible reference to use on a busy clinical shift.

We will cover how to perform an array of nerve blocks. This reference, along with guided practice, can help emergency physicians develop competency with as many of these procedures as possible.

Our editorial team hopes this guide serves you and your patients well, as you provide better, safer, definitive pain control in the emergency department.

— *The Editors-in-Chief*

TABLE OF CONTENTS

EMRA members: Access a digital version with videos and bonus content via the QR code.

INTRODUCTION

Approach to Analgesia 9
Leland K. Perice, MD | The Warren Alpert Medical School of Brown University

Local Anesthetic (LA) Choice 9
Leland K. Perice, MD | The Warren Alpert Medical School of Brown University

Dosing 10
Leland K. Perice, MD | The Warren Alpert Medical School of Brown University

Risks of Regional Anesthesia (RA) 11
Leland K. Perice, MD | The Warren Alpert Medical School of Brown University

Local Anesthetic Systemic Toxicity (LAST)..13
Leland K. Perice, MD | The Warren Alpert Medical School of Brown University
Rachael Duncan, PharmD, BCPS, BCCCP | Heart of the Rockies Regional Medical Center

HEAD AND NECK

*All authored by Marc L. Martel, MD | Hennepin Healthcare and
University of Minnesota Medical School*

Superficial Cervical Plexus Block 16
Greater Auricular Nerve Block...18
Occipital Nerve Block...20
Supraorbital Nerve Block 22
Infraorbital Nerve Block..24
Mental Nerve Block...26

TORSO

Pectoralis (PECS) I and II Plane Block 30
Robert F. Reardon, MD | Hennepin Healthcare and University of Minnesota Medical School

Serratus Anterior Plane Block 32
Alexis LaPietra, DO | St. Joseph's Regional Medical Center
Katherine Vlasica, DO | St. Joseph's Regional Medical Center

Erector Spinae Plane Block 34
Andrew J. Goldsmith, MD, MBA | Brigham and Women's Hospital & Harvard Medical School
Joseph Stegeman, MD | Harvard Affiliated Emergency Medicine Residency

Transverse Abdominus Plane (TAP) Block 36
Marc L. Martel, MD | Hennepin Healthcare & University of Minnesota Medical School

UPPER EXTREMITY

Interscalene Brachial Plexus Block 40
Arun D. Nagdev, MD | Highland Hospital & University of California, San Francisco
Daniel Mantuani, MD, MPH | Highland Hospital & University of California, San Francisco

Supraclavicular Brachial Plexus Block 42
Arun D. Nagdev, MD | Highland Hospital & University of California, San Francisco
Daniel Mantuani, MD, MPH | Highland Hospital & University of California, San Francisco

Suprascapular Nerve Block 44
Marc L. Martel, MD | Hennepin Healthcare & University of Minnesota Medical School

Axillary Brachial Plexus Block 46
Robert F. Reardon, MD | Hennepin Healthcare & University of Minnesota Medical School

Ulnar Nerve Block 48
Alexis LaPietra, DO | St. Joseph's Regional Medical Center
Igor Middlebrook, DO, MS | University of North Carolina Health Wayne

Radial Nerve Block 50
Alexis LaPietra, DO | St. Joseph's Regional Medical Center
Igor Middlebrook, DO, MS | University of North Carolina Health Wayne

Median Nerve Block 52
Kristin H. Dwyer, MD, MPH | The Warren Alpert Medical School of Brown University

Landmark-Based Hand Block 54
Kristin H. Dwyer, MD, MPH | The Warren Alpert Medical School of Brown University

LOWER EXTREMITY

Periscapular Nerve Group (PENG) Block 60
Andrew J. Goldsmith, MD, MBA | Brigham and Women's Hospital & Harvard Medical School
Joseph Stegeman, MD | Harvard Affiliated Emergency Medicine Residency

Transgluteal Sciatic Nerve Block 62
Andrew J. Goldsmith, MD, MBA | Brigham and Women's Hospital & Harvard Medical School
Nicole M. Duggan, MD | Brigham and Women's Hospital & Harvard Medical School

Infrainguinal Fascia Iliaca Plane Block 64
Arun D. Nagdev, MD | Highland Hospital, University of California, San Francisco
Daniel Mantuani, MD, MPH | Highland Hospital

Saphenous Nerve/Adductor Canal Block 66
Robert F. Reardon, MD | Hennepin Healthcare & University of Minnesota Medical School

Distal Sciatic Nerve Block in Popliteal Fossa 68
Andrew J. Goldsmith, MD, MBA | Brigham and Women's Hospital & Harvard Medical School
Nicole M. Duggan, MD | Brigham and Women's Hospital & Harvard Medical School

Ankle Block 70
Kristin H. Dwyer, MD, MPH | The Warren Alpert Medical School of Brown University

Distal Tibial Nerve 72
Arun D. Nagdev, MD | Highland Hospital, University of California, San Francisco
Daniel Mantuani, MD, MPH | Highland Hospital

OTHER MSK PROCEDURES

Hematoma Block for Humerus Fractures 76
Ramnik Dhaliwal, MD, JD | Carepoint Health

Hematoma Block for Ankle Fractures 77
Ramnik Dhaliwal, MD, JD | Carepoint Health

Hematoma Block for Wrist Fractures 78
Ramnik Dhaliwal, MD, JD | Carepoint Health

Trigger Point Injection: Thoracic and Lumbar Muscles 80
Aaron Schaffner, MD | Baptist Medical Center East
Donald E. Stader III, MD | Carepoint Health

Trigger Point Injection: Cervical and Trapezius Muscles 82
Aaron Schaffner, MD | Baptist Medical Center East
Donald E. Stader III, MD | Carepoint Health

Knee Injection 84
Arun D. Nagdev, MD | Highland Hospital, University of California, San Francisco
Alan C. Taylor, MD | University of Tennessee Health Science Center
Emily Lovallo, MD, | University of Pittsburgh
Brian Johnson, MD, MPH | Valley Medical Center - University of Washington
Daniel Mantuani, MD, MPH | Highland Hospital & University of California, San Francisco

Shoulder Injection 86
Arun D. Nagdev, MD | Highland Hospital, University of California, San Francisco
Tony A. Downs, MD | University of Tennessee Health Science Center

Hip Injection 88
Arun D. Nagdev, MD | Highland Hospital, University of California, San Francisco
Marcin Byra, DO | University of Tennessee Health Science Center
Daniel Mantuani, MD, MPH | Highland Hospital & University of California, San Francisco
Caitlin Bailey, MD | Highland Hospital & University of California, San Francisco

ADMINSTRATION/OPERATIONS

What Is Advanced Analgesia 92
Donald E. Stader III, MD | Carepoint Health

Evidence of Benefit 92
Leland K. Perice, MD | The Warren Alpert Medical School of Brown University

How to Implement Regional Anesthesia Training 93
(All authors from Highland Hospital & University of California, San Francisco)
Arun D. Nagdev, MD
Kaitlen Howell, MD
Akash Desai, MD
David Martin, MD
Daniel Mantuani, MD, MPH

Reimbursement 97
Aaron Schaffner, MD | Baptist Medical Center East

APPENDIX

References 100
Index 111

INTRODUCTION

Approach to Regional Anesthesia
- Endorsed by American College of Surgeons as best practice in the management of trauma patients
- Emergency department (ED) benefits:
  - Decreased length of stay
  - Reduced need for procedural sedation
  - Reduction in opioid requirements
  - Increased overall patient satisfaction compared to other methods of pain control
  - May decrease mortality for hip and rib fractures
- Ultrasound-guided regional anesthesia (UGRA)
  - Higher success rate than landmark-based RA
  - Decreased time of onset
  - Lower anesthetic volume required
  - Faster block performance time
  - Decreased rate of complications

Local Anesthetic Choice
- It is important to know the specific characteristics of the commonly used local anesthetics (LA) in the ED, as they have different onset times, duration of action, and risk profiles.

Mechanism of Action
- Reversible inhibition of sodium ion influx into nerve fibers, blocking depolarization and overall transmission of pain along the nerve
  - Different LAs have differing degrees of duration of action and toxicity

Time to Onset
- Dependent upon each LA's:
  - Lipid solubility
  - pKA
  - Protein binding
  - Concentration
- Specific agent choice and concentration determine how fast LA diffuses into nerves and surrounding tissues
  - 2% lidocaine faster onset of action than 1% lidocaine
  - Ropivacaine, bupivacaine, levobupivacaine slower onset of action than "fast onset" LAs such as lidocaine, mepivacaine, chloroprocaine

Classes of Anesthetics
- Amides: Amide LAs can be remembered as they have 2 i's
  - Lidocaine
  - Bupivacaine
  - Ropivacaine

- Esters (used if allergy to amides)
  - Chloroprocaine
  - Procaine
  - Tetracaine
- If allergic to both amides and esters, consider 1% diphenhydramine for simple procedures (such as laceration repairs)
  - Scant evidence for use as a substitute for larger plane or nerve blocks

Local Anesthetic Dosing & Maximum Dose

- Supratherapeutic doses may result in Local Anesthetic Systemic Toxicity (LAST)
  - Significant morbidity and mortality
  - See p. 13 and foldout back cover
- Maximum doses based on ideal body weight

Local Anesthetic Maximum Bolus Doses in Regional Anesthesia

Local Anesthetic	Max Dose (mg/kg)	50 kg (mL)	60 kg (mL)	70 kg (mL)	80 kg (mL)	90 kg (mL)	100 kg (mL)	Half-life Additional Considerations
Bupivacaine 0.25% (2.5 mg/mL)	2 mg /kg+	40 mL 100 mg	48 mL 120 mg	56 mL 140 mg	64 mL 160 mg	70 mL 175 mg*		• 4-8 hrs • Contraindicated in pregnancy • More likely to cause cardiac toxicity
Bupivacaine 0.5% (5 mg/mL)		20 mL 100 mg	24 mL 120 mg	28 mL 140 mg	32 mL 160 mg	35 mL 175 mg*		
Ropivacaine 0.2% (2 mg/mL)	3 mg /kg	75 mL 150 mg	90 mL 180 mg	105 mL 210 mg	120 mL 240 mg	135 mL 270 mg	150 mL* 300 mg	• 4-10 hrs • Less cardiotoxic than bupivacaine making it safer for high-dose, high-volume blocks
Ropivacaine 0.5% (5 mg/mL)		30 mL 150 mg	36 mL 180 mg	42 mL 210 mg	48 mL 240 mg	54 mL 270 mg	60 mL* 300 mg	
Lidocaine 1% (10 mg/mL)	4 mg /kg	20 mL 200 mg	24 mL 240 mg	28 mL 280 mg	30 mL* 300 mg			• 1-4 hrs • Do not repeat within 2 hrs • Ideal for shorter blocks
Lidocaine 2% (20 mg/mL)		10 mL 200 mg	12 mL 240 mg	14 mL 280 mg	15 mL* 300 mg			
Lidocaine 1% w/ epi (10 mg/mL)	7 mg /kg	35 mL 350 mg	42 mL 420 mg	49 mL 490 mg	50 mL* 500 mg			• 2-6 hrs • Relative contraindication for penile blocks

+Bupivacaine is associated with a greater risk of cardiac toxicity, likely because it readily crosses lipid layers and inhibits the sodium channels in the heart. As such, the safe doses of bupivacaine are much lower than that of the other anesthetics used in the ED.

*Do not exceed maximum recommended dose regardless of weight

Dosing Adjustment Considerations
CAUTION: Dosing charts are best applied to healthy patients; consider lower maximum doses in physiologically frail patients

Decrease dosage and consider consulting pharmacy if:
- Renal dysfunction
- Extremes of age
- Hepatic dysfunction (reduces clearance of LA)
- Advanced heart failure (CHF reduces clearance of LA)
- Pregnancy (increases nerve susceptibility to LA)

Additives to Prolong Duration
CAUTION: Significant debate and no clear consensus in the literature
- Dexamethasone (commonly used in EDs)
  - A Cochrane review has shown perineural dexamethasone to increase anesthetic efficiency up to 8 hrs for doses ranging from 4-10 mg
  - Most effective; can prolong RA up to 6-8 hrs when added to long-acting LA such as ropivacaine or bupivacaine
  - Minimal adverse effects
  - Commonly stocked in the ED
- Epinephrine (commonly used in EDs)
  - Increases therapeutic margin for short-acting LA such as lidocaine
  - Can decrease neural blood flow, which can increase risk of neurotoxicity
    - Not proven to be clinically significant risk
  - Traditionally used as marker of intravascular injection
    - Less pertinent when ultrasound is used
- Midazolam
- Clonidine
- Dexmedetomidine
- Buprenorphine
- Sodium bicarbonate

Risks of Regional Anesthesia
CAUTION: Thoroughly understand risks and benefits before performing a block
- Complications associated with RA
  - Infection
  - Bleeding
  - Neurologic injury
  - Injury to adjacent structures
  - Local anesthetic systemic toxicity (LAST)
  - Vascular injury
  - Diaphragmatic paralysis
  - Horner syndrome
  - Pneumothorax

- Factors that increase risk for mechanical trauma (from needle) or LA toxicity (both local and systemic)
  - Comorbidities
  - Extremes of age
  - Location of block
  - LA agent used
  - Concentration
  - Volume/amount of LA used

Safety Protocols

- Please use local hospital guidelines
- Cardiac monitoring (heart rate, blood pressure, pulse oximetry)
  - Exception is low volume or distal to elbow and knee
- Drugs to treat LAST
  - Intralipid 20%
  - Benzodiazepines and antiepileptic agents for seizures
  - ACLS drugs for cardiac arrest
- IV access for all high-volume blocks, blocks with risk of vascular injection or LAST
- Rapid access to emergent airway equipment

Infection

- Use basic infection control
  - Skin disinfection and personal protective equipment (PPE)
  - Probe covers
- Refer to local infection control guidelines and standards at your institution

Nerve Injury

- Peripheral Nerve Injury (PNI), defined as a motor deficit that persists > 72 hrs, is rare: 2-4/10,000 procedures
  - Patient risk factors associated with higher chance of PNI: diabetes, peripheral vascular disease, hypertension, smoking, vasculitis
- Majority resolve within weeks; 99.9% of these peripheral neuropathies resolve within a year
- Injury mechanism: direct needle trauma and/or intraneural injection
- Recommend extra-neural anesthetic deposition or "stay away from the nerve" technique to reduce direct mechanical trauma from malpositioned needle tip
- Factors/techniques used to help reduce the risk of neural injury include:
  - **Operator competency:** Previous US-based procedural skills. Specific US techniques and methods that improve needle visualization include:
    - **Hydrolocation:** Inject small amount of normal saline to produce a small anechoic window, allowing better needle tip visualization
    - **Hydrodissection:** Inject small volumes of saline to open fascial planes to define correct location of anesthetic

- Decreased angle of needle insertion/insonation: Decreasing the angle between needle and probe helps visualize the needle
- Use echogenic needles
- Monitor symptoms such as electrical or shock-type pain, paresthesias, or significant pain with injection

Needle selection
- Use short tip/blunt tip needles when performing US-guided nerve blocks
- Use US-guided specific block needles: blunt, often serrated tip (can improve US visualization)
- Alternative: Quincke spinal needles
- Not recommended: long bevel/sharp tip needles commonly used in ED for local skin infiltration

Needle tips
- Needles with blunt bevels generally considered safer to use with nerve blocks
  - Less likely to cause unintentional cutting or trauma
  - Bevel is slanting edge at tip of needle (A Bevel is sharpest; C is most blunt)

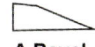 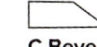

LOCAL ANESTHETIC SYSTEMIC TOXICITY (LAST)

- **Life-threatening adverse reaction**
- Generally seen with accidental intravascular injection or excess dosage
- Risk varies according to block
  - Generally, higher risk with blocks that occur closer to large blood vessels or involve large volumes
  - Debate exists between experts on increased risk of LAST from thoracic plane blocks; several experts advocate for using lower than maximum doses for thoracic plane blocks
- Mechanism unclear but believed to be caused by blockade of sodium channels in CNS and cardiac tissue
  - Blocked sodium channels in cortical neurons results in seizures and respiratory arrest
- Symptoms of LAST
  - Generally progressive; see **Figure 1**, p. 14
  - If symptoms begin, immediately stop injection/infusion and consider intralipid
    - Bupivacaine carries more risk, due to increased cardiac toxicity compared to other LAs
    - Ropivacaine is generally considered less cardiotoxic than bupivacaine

- Treatment of LAST (see back cover)
  - Standard care for seizures and/or cardiac arrest
  - Lipid emulsion therapy with intralipid 20%
  - Dosing based on ideal body weight
    - **Bolus:** 1-1.5 mL/kg over 1 min (typical 100 mL)
      - Can repeat every 3 min up to a total dose of 3 mL/kg
    - **Infusion:** 0.25 mL/kg/min (typical 20 mL/min)
      - Continue until hemodynamically stable for at least 10 min
      - Can increase infusion to 0.5 mL/kg/min if BP worsens
  - Equipment and supplies needed to recognize and treat LAST should be in place before any procedure
    - Cardiac monitoring
    - IV access
    - Rapidly accessible intralipid (with dosing instructions included in lipid rescue kit)
  - Delay in the decision to administer intralipid can lead to morbidity and mortality
    - Essentially no downside to treating with intralipid if LAST is suspected
    - See lipid rescue algorithm, foldout back cover

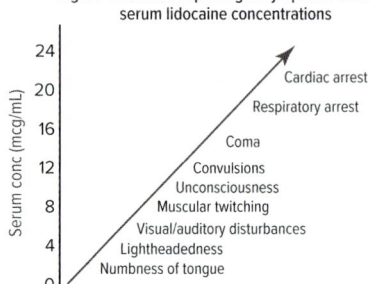

Figure 1. Relationship of signs/symptoms of toxicity to serum lidocaine concentrations

HEAD AND NECK

Superficial Cervical Plexus Block 16
Greater Auricular Nerve Block 18
Occipital Nerve Block 20
Supraorbital Nerve Block 22
Infraorbital Nerve Block 24
Mental Nerve Block 26

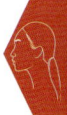

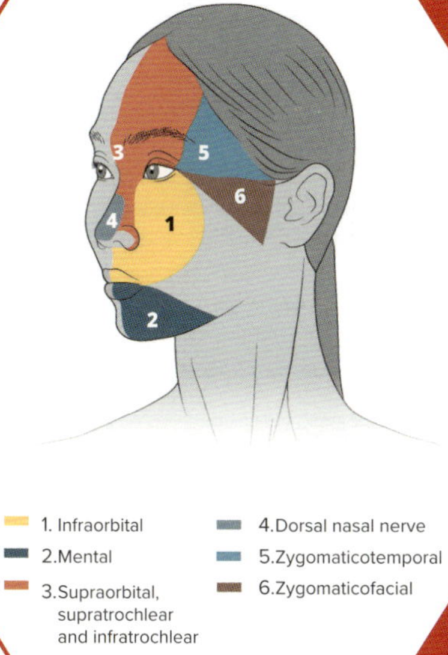

1. Infraorbital
2. Mental
3. Supraorbital, supratrochlear and infratrochlear
4. Dorsal nasal nerve
5. Zygomaticotemporal
6. Zygomaticofacial

SUPERFICIAL CERVICAL PLEXUS BLOCK

Materials *(adapt to patient, clinician, and site-specific factors/availability)*

Probe	High-frequency linear probe
Needle	50 mm, 22 G blunt tip needle Hyperechoic block needle preferred, tubing optional
Volume of anesthetic	5 mL
Other	5-10 mL syringe Skin prep and PPE *Optional: 1-2 mL 1% lidocaine in separate syringe for skin wheal*

Region of Analgesia
Anesthetizes the sensory branches of the C2, C3, and C4 nerve roots as well as the lesser occipital, transverse cervical, and greater auricular, supraclavicular nerves (not to be confused with supraclavicular brachial plexus block). Anesthesia is achieved in the area of the anterior and lateral neck, including the inferior and posterior aspects of the auricle and extends caudally to cover the area of the clavicle. There is no motor involvement (**Figure 1**).

Indications	Contraindications
• Clavicle fracture • Placement of internal jugular central lines • Inferior ear lacerations/infections • Drainage of anterior/lateral neck abscesses • Burn management	• Allergy to local anesthetic • Overlying infection • Anticoagulation (relative) • O_2 dependence and/or single lung on side of block (relative)

Patient Positioning
- Supine, with head turned to contralateral side
- May also be performed with patient in lateral decubitus position (**Figure 2**)

Procedure
1. Sterilize field per local guidelines.
2. **Place** probe at posterolateral aspect of sternocleidomastoid (SCM) muscle in a transverse orientation.
3. **Identify** SCM at level of thyroid cartilage, the lateral aspect of SCM with anterior scalene muscles in view (deep) and the carotid artery. Target is the plane between SCM and levator scapulae muscle layers.
4. Using an in-plane approach, **direct** the needle tip to be under SCM fascial layer at posterolateral border.
5. Once a homogeneous anechoic stripe is observed between SCM and levator scapulae muscle, **inject** 5 mL anesthetic.

Head and Neck

Figure 1. Region of analgesia

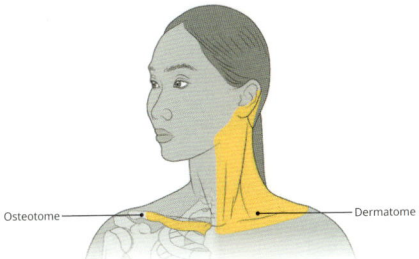

Osteotome — Dermatome

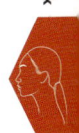

Figure 2 (left): Probe placement
Figure 3 (below): Ultrasound anatomy

1. Sternocleidomastoid muscle
2. Cervical Plexus branches
3. Carotid artery
4. Anterior scalene muscles
5. Internal jugular vein

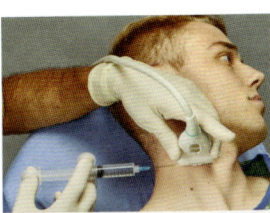

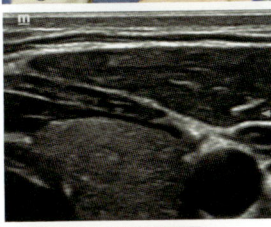

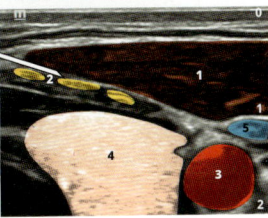

Pearls and Pitfalls

- This is a very superficial block.
- Always note the location of the carotid artery.
- Always aspirate to avoid intravascular injection.
- Although brachial plexus involvement and phrenic nerve paralysis are rare, consider avoiding in patients with severe respiratory compromise.
- Increasing volumes over 5 mL, especially over 10 mL, increases risk of Horner syndrome from LA spread to the deep cervical plexus.

GREATER AURICULAR NERVE BLOCK

Materials *(adapt to patient, clinician, and site-specific factors/availability)*

Probe	High-frequency linear probe
Needle	50 mm, 22 G blunt tip needle
	Hyperechoic block needle preferred, tubing optional
Volume of anesthetic	3-5 mL
Other	10 mL syringe
	Skin prep and PPE
	Optional: 1-2 mL 1% lidocaine in separate syringe for skin wheal

Region of Analgesia

Anesthetizes the helix, concha, and lobule of the auricle through its innervation of the C2 and C3 nerve roots. There is no motor involvement (**Figure 1**).

Indications	Contraindications
• Lacerations of auricle	• Allergy to local anesthetic
• Abscess of the auricle	• Overlying infection

Patient Positioning

- Supine, with head turned to contralateral side
- May be performed with patient in lateral decubitus position (**Figure 2**)

Procedure

1. Sterilize field per local guidelines.
2. **Place** probe at posterolateral aspect of the sternocleidomastoid (SCM) muscle in a transverse orientation.
3. **Identify** the SCM at the level of the thyroid cartilage, the lateral aspect of the SCM with the levator scapulae muscle in view (deep) and the carotid artery.
4. **Scan** cranially along the SCM until the probe is approximately 3-5 cm inferior to the ear and the greater auricular nerve is identified superficially, near the angle of the mandible.
5. Using an in-plane approach, **direct** your needle tip to be adjacent to the greater auricular nerve.
6. After aspiration, **inject** 3-5 mL anesthetic adjacent to the nerve.

Figure 1. Region of analgesia

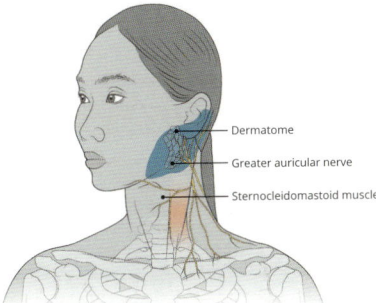
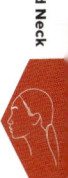

Head and Neck

- Dermatome
- Greater auricular nerve
- Sternocleidomastoid muscle

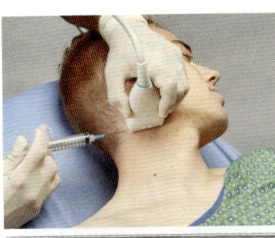

Figure 2 (left): Probe placement
Figure 3 (below): Ultrasound anatomy

1. Greater auricular nerve
2. Sternocleidomastoid muscle
3. Levator scapulae muscle

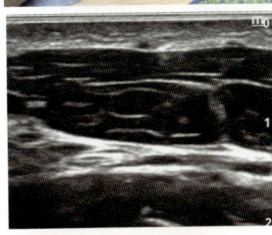
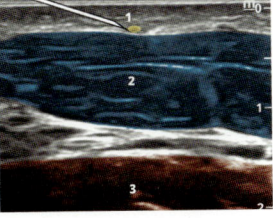

Pearls and Pitfalls

- Keep your needle angle shallow, as this is a very superficial block.

OCCIPITAL NERVE BLOCK

Materials *(adapt to patient, clinician, and site-specific factors/availability)*

Needle	25-27 G, 1.5" long beveled/sharp tip needle
Volume of anesthetic	3-5 mL per side; 6-10 mL if bilateral block performed
Other	5-10 mL syringe Skin prep and PPE

Region of Analgesia

Anesthetizes the posterior scalp from the vertex to the level of the occipital protuberance through its innervation of C2 nerve root. There is no motor involvement (**Figure 1**).

Indications	Contraindications
• Occipital scalp lacerations and abscess • Occipital and tension headaches	• Allergy to local anesthetic • Overlying infection • Skull fracture or defect • Anticoagulation (relative)

Patient Positioning

■ Prone or seated on gurney with head flexed forward, facing away from operator (**Figures 3-4**)

Procedure

1. Sterilize field per local guidelines.
2. **Palpate** occipital protuberance. The occipital nerve lies medial to palpable occipital artery, approximately 1/3 the distance laterally, from midline to mastoid.
3. **Direct** needle toward occiput from below. **Aspirate** first, then **inject** local anesthesia in fan-like distribution.
4. Alternatively, **inject** local anesthesia transversely from medial to lateral, overlying area where nerve originates.

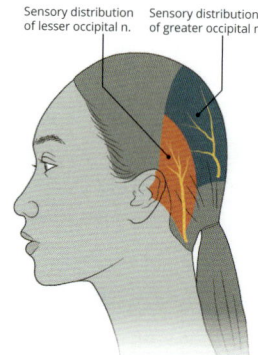

Figure 1: Region of analgesia

Figure 2. Anatomy

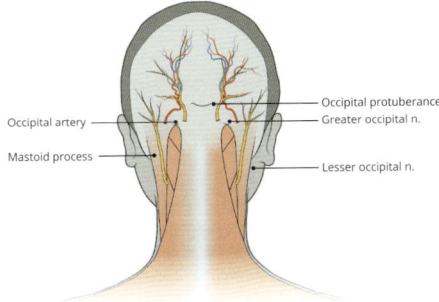
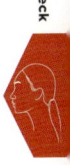

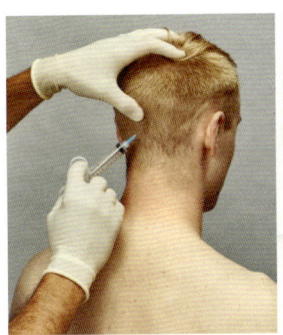

Figure 3: Needle placement, greater occipital nerve block

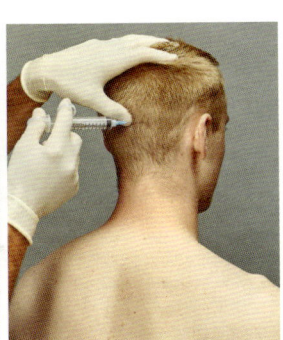

Figure 4: Needle placement, lesser occipital nerve block

Pearls and Pitfalls

- This is a superficial block.
- Evidence of benefit in migraine, tension and occipital neuralgia-type headaches.

SUPRAORBITAL NERVE BLOCK

Materials *(adapt to patient, clinician, and site-specific factors/availability)*

Probe	Optional; high-frequency linear probe if US is used
Needle	25-27 G, 1.5" long beveled/sharp tip needle
Volume of anesthetic	1-3 mL per side; 2-6 mL if bilateral block performed
Other	5-10 mL syringe Skin prep and PPE

Region of Analgesia
Anesthetizes the forehead, eyebrow, upper eyelid, and the anterior, superior portion of the nose through its innervation of the ophthalmic nerve (V1). There is no motor involvement (**Figure 1**).

Indications	Contraindications
• Laceration repair of the eyebrow and forehead • Abscess and/or burn management	• Allergy to local anesthetic • Injection through infected tissue (relative) • Pre-existing nerve injury (relative)

Patient Positioning
- Supine or seated on gurney

Procedure
Ultrasound-Guided approach
1. Sterilize field per local guidelines.
2. With patient's eye closed, **place** ultrasound probe over the medial aspect of the supraorbital rim.
3. The supraorbital notch is identified as the indent in the bone.
4. **Advance** the needle inferior to superior, using an out-of-plane approach.
5. After negative aspiration, **inject** local anesthesia in the region of the supraorbital notch, under direct visualization.

Anatomic (landmark) approach
1. Sterilize field per local guidelines.
2. **Palpate** supraorbital foramen on the orbital rim ~ 2 cm from midline.
3. **Advance** the needle transversely, superficially over the orbital rim.
4. After negative aspiration, **inject** local anesthetic linearly while slowly **removing** the needle back toward the entrance in the skin.

Figure 1. Region of analgesia

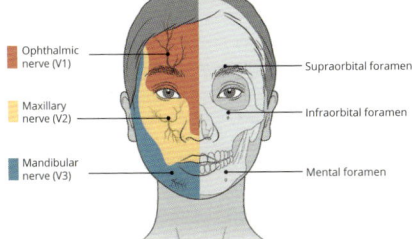
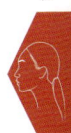

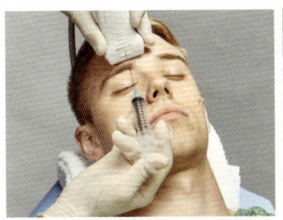

Figure 2: Needle placement with ultrasound   Figure 3: Needle placement (no ultrasound)

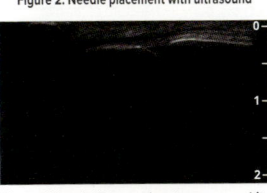
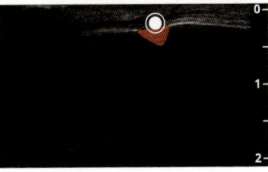

Figure 4 (above): Ultrasound anatomy; supraorbital nerve foramen (above, right)

Pearls and Pitfalls

- Although ultrasound guidance is feasible, this block is most commonly performed using palpation of anatomic landmarks.
- Particularly when used for laceration repair, it is crucial to document function (or absence) of the supraorbital nerve prior to blockade.
- This technique will commonly block both the supratrochlear and supraorbital nerves.

INFRAORBITAL NERVE BLOCK

Materials *(adapt to patient, clinician, and site-specific factors/availability)*

Probe	Optional; high-frequency linear probe, if US is used
Needle	25-27 G, 1.5" long beveled/sharp tip needle
Volume of anesthetic	1-3 mL per side; 2-6 mL if bilateral block performed
Other	5-10 mL syringe Skin prep and PPE

Region of Analgesia

Anesthetizes the cutaneous and mucosal surfaces of the upper lip, lateral nose, and lower portion of the eyelid through the infraorbital nerve of the terminal branch of the maxillary nerve (V2). There is no motor involvement (**Figure 1**).

Indications	Contraindications
• Laceration repair of the lip and cheek • Abscess and burn management	• Allergy to local anesthetic • Injection through infected tissue (relative) • Pre-existing nerve injury (relative)

Patient Positioning
- Supine or seated on gurney

Procedure
Ultrasound-guided approach
1. Sterilize field per local guidelines.
2. **Place** probe over maxilla, ~1 cm below lower orbit.
3. Infraorbital notch is the indent in hyperechoic, bony architecture of maxilla.
4. **Advance** needle inferior to superior, using an out-of-plane approach.
5. After negative aspiration, **inject** anesthetic in region of the infraorbital notch, under direct visualization.

Anatomic (landmark) approach

Intraoral
1. Using nondominant hand, palpate infraorbital foramen on cutaneous surface, below orbital rim. Using nondominant thumb and index finger, lift upper lip.
2. Palpate infraorbital foramen intraorally above area of lateral incisor.
3. Insert needle in gingival mucosa, superiorly toward foramen.
4. After negative aspiration, inject anesthetic in region of foramen.

Extraoral
1. Sterilize field per local guidelines.
2. Palpate infraorbital foramen.
3. Insert needle below foramen, directed with slight cephalic approach.
4. Avoid direct penetration of foramen.
5. After negative aspiration, inject desired anesthetic in region of foramen.

Figure 1. Region of analgesia

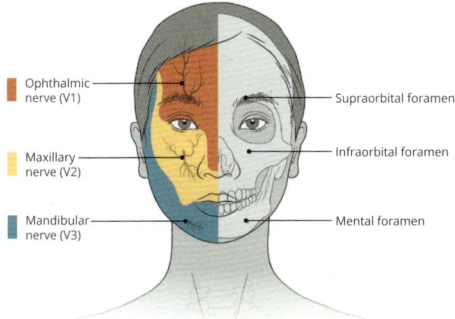

- Ophthalmic nerve (V1)
- Maxillary nerve (V2)
- Mandibular nerve (V3)
- Supraorbital foramen
- Infraorbital foramen
- Mental foramen

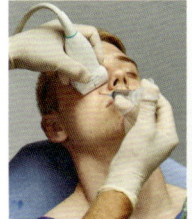 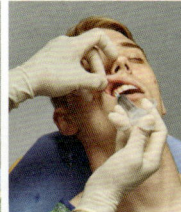 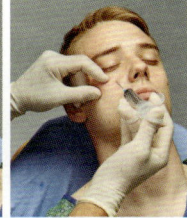

Figure 2: Probe placement (above, left); superficial landmarks (intraoral - above, center; extraoral - above, right)

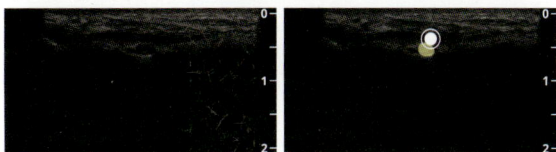

Figure 3: Ultrasound anatomy (above, left); infraorbital nerve foramen (above, right)

Pearls and Pitfalls

- Although ultrasound guidance is feasible, this block is most commonly performed using palpation of anatomic landmarks.
- Particularly when used for laceration repair, it is crucial to document function and/or the absence function of the infraorbital nerve.

MENTAL NERVE BLOCK

Materials *(adapt to patient, clinician, and site-specific factors/availability)*

Probe	Optional; high-frequency linear probe, if US is used
Needle	25-27 G, 1.5" long beveled/sharp tip needle
Volume of anesthetic	1-3 mL per side; 2-6 mL if bilateral block performed
Other	5-10 mL syringe Skin prep and PPE

Region of Analgesia

Anesthetizes the cutaneous and mucosal surfaces of the lower lip and chin through the mental nerve branch of the inferior alveolar nerve of the mandibular nerve (V3). There is no motor involvement (**Figure 1**).

Indications	Contraindications
• Laceration repair of the lip and chin • Abscess and burn management	• Allergy to local anesthetic • Injection through infected tissue (relative) • Pre-existing nerve injury (relative)

Patient Positioning

- Supine or seated on gurney

Procedure
Ultrasound-guided approach

1. Sterilize field per local guidelines.
2. **Place** probe over mandible, ~1 cm above lower border, ~3 cm lateral of midline.
3. The mental foramen is the indent in the bony architecture of the mandible.
4. **Advance** needle inferior to superior, using an out-of-plane approach.
5. After negative aspiration, **inject** anesthetic in the region of the mental foramen, under direct visualization.

Anatomic (landmark) approach

Intraoral

1. With nondominant hand, palpate mental foramen on cutaneous surface on lower mandible, simultaneously retracting lower lip. Palpate foramen intraorally above area of lower, first premolar.
2. Insert needle in gingival mucosa, directed inferiorly toward foramen.
3. After negative aspiration, inject local anesthetic in the region of foramen.

Extraoral

1. Sterilize field per local guidelines.
2. Palpate mental foramen (in line with pupil and supraorbital/infraorbital foramen).
3. Insert needle lateral to foramen, directed medially.
4. After negative aspiration, inject local anesthetic in region of foramen.

Figure 1. Region of analgesia

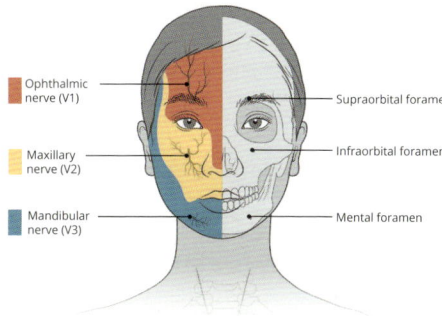
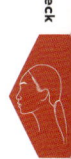

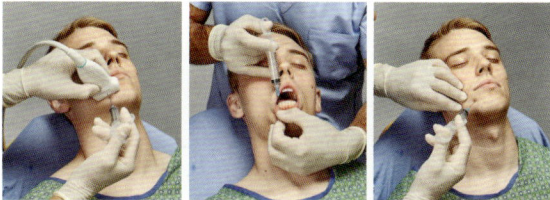

Figure 2: Probe placement (above, left); superficial landmarks (intraoral - above, center; extraoral - above, right)

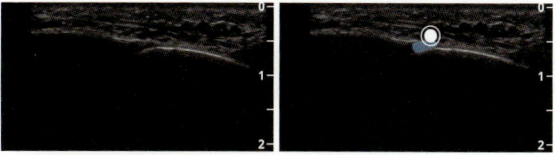

Figure 3: Ultrasound anatomy (above, left; mental nerve foramen (above, right)

Pearls and Pitfalls

- Although ultrasound guidance is feasible, this block is most commonly performed using palpation of anatomic landmarks.
- Particularly when used for laceration repair, it is crucial to document function or absence of function of the mental nerve prior to blockade.
- Avoid direct penetration of the mental foramen.

Head and Neck

TORSO

Pectoralis (PECS) I and II Plane Block 30
Serratus Anterior Plane Block 32
Erector Spinae Plane Block 34
Transabdominal Plane (TAP) Block 36

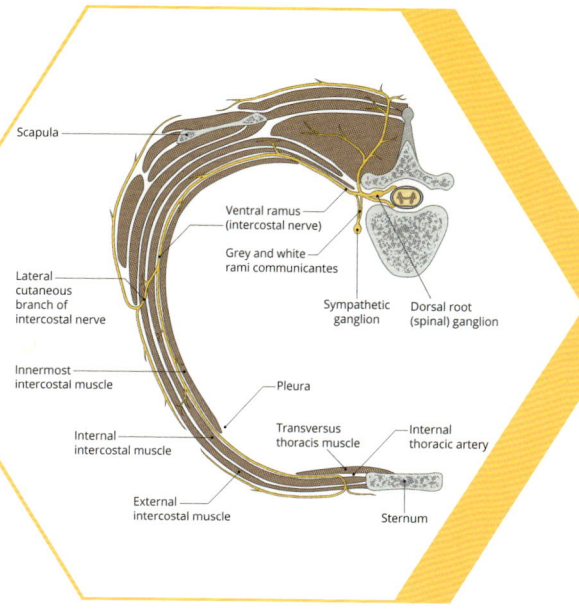

PECTORALIS (PECS) I AND II PLANE BLOCK

Materials *(adapt to patient, clinician, and site-specific factors/availability)*

Probe	High-frequency linear probe
Needle	50–100 mm, 22 G blunt tip needle Hyperechoic block needle with tubing
Volume of anesthetic	10 mL for PECS I; 20 mL for PECS II
Other	30 mL syringe, 10 mL sterile saline (for hydrodissection) Skin prep and PPE *Optional: 1-2 mL lidocaine in separate syringe for skin wheal*

Region of Analgesia
- **PECS I:** Anesthetizes the superior and lateral portions of breast and pectoralis major/minor muscles through medial and lateral pectoral nerves.
- **PECS II:** Anesthetizes the entire breast, axillary region, and anterior chest (T2-T6 nerve roots) through long thoracic, thoracodorsal, intercostal nerves.
- May affect adduction of affected side's arm, but rarely (PECS I) (**Figure 1**).

Indications	Contraindications
• Breast and pacemaker post operative pain relief	• Allergy to local anesthetic
• Anterior and/or lateral rib fractures (PECS II)	• Overlying infection
• Breast and axillary (PECS II) abscesses	• Anticoagulation (relative contraindication)
• Chest wall lacerations and burns (PECS I or II)	
• Thoracostomy (PECS II)	

Patient Positioning
- Supine, with head turned away from affected side and operator at head of bed

Procedure
1. Sterilize field per local guidelines.
2. **Place** probe in sagittal/oblique plane, inferior to clavicle, at lateral portion of pectoralis major, level of 4th rib.
3. **Identify** sonoanatomy seen as horizontal tissue planes — pectoralis major muscle, pectoralis minor muscle, serratus anterior muscle, ribs (2nd/3rd or 3rd/4th), and lung.
4. To block both PECS I and II: Using in-plane approach from cephalad to caudad, **advance** needle tip into plane between serratus anterior muscle and pectoralis minor muscle (PECS II block).
5. After negative aspiration, **confirm** placement using hydrodissection to open planes. Once confirmed, **inject** 20 mL anesthetic (PECS II).
6. If also performing PECS I block, **retract** until needle tip is between pectoralis major and minor muscles.
7. After negative aspiration, **confirm** needle placement using hydrodissection to open the planes. Once confirmed, **inject** 10 mL anesthetic.

Figure 1. Innervation of the anterior/lateral chest wall and breast

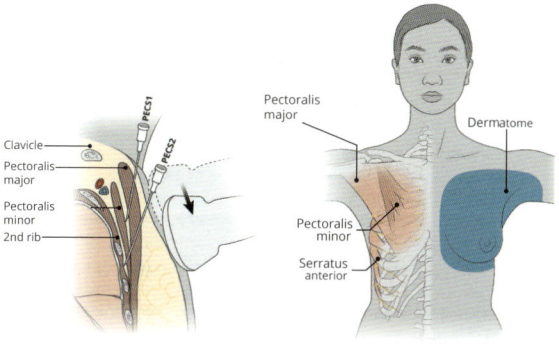

1. Pectoralis major 2. PECS I 3. Pectoralis minor 4. PECS II 5. Serratus Anterior
6. Rib 7. Pleura

Figure 2 (below, left): Probe placement
Figure 3 (below, center and right): Ultrasound anatomy

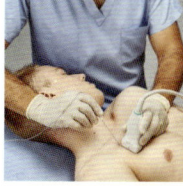
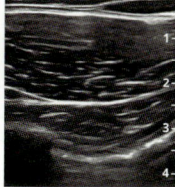
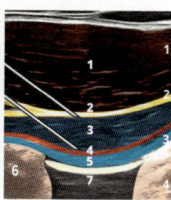

Pearls and Pitfalls

- Increasing volume (by dilution of LA), while staying within safe dose, can enhance spread and efficacy of block.
- PECS I & II are performed together with one needle-stick for breast and anterior chest soft tissue anesthesia.
- Debate exists between experts on increased risk of LAST from thoracic plane blocks. Several experts advocate for using lower than maximum doses.

SERRATUS ANTERIOR PLANE BLOCK

Materials *(adapt to patient, clinician, and site-specific factors/availability)*

Probe	High-frequency linear probe
Needle	50-100 mm, 22 G blunt tip needle
	Hyperechoic block needle with tubing
Volume of anesthetic	20-40 mL anesthetic (dilute if needed; split dose between 2 syringes as needed)
Other	30-50 mL syringe, 10 mL sterile saline (for hydrodissection)
	Skin prep and PPE
	Optional: 1-2 mL 1% lidocaine in separate syringe for skin wheal

Region of Analgesia
Anesthetizes the T2–T9 dermatomes of the ipsilateral hemithorax through the lateral cutaneous nerves, long thoracic nerve, and thoracodorsal nerve, relieving pain in the anterior and lateral chest wall. It is possible to have a temporary wing scapula as a result of this block (**Figure 1**).

Indications	Contraindications
• Anterior and/or lateral rib fractures	• Allergy to local anesthetic
• Thoracostomy insertion	• Overlying infection
• Complex chest lacerations and abscesses	• Anticoagulation (relative contraindication)
• Chest wall burns	
• Chest wall herpes zoster rash	

Patient Positioning
- Supine or lateral decubitus position with injured side up, with arm above or perpendicular to torso, allowing for probe and operator at site of injection

Procedure
1. Sterilize field per local guidelines.
2. **Place** transducer in a transverse plane at the midaxillary line at the 4th or 5th rib.
3. **Identify** ribs with underlying pleura. The first muscle layer above ribs is the serratus anterior. At the level of mid-axillary line, the second beak-shaped muscle layer above the serratus muscles is the latissimus dorsi muscle.
4. Using an in-line needle approach, **direct** the needle to the fascial layer between the serratus anterior and latissimus dorsi.
5. After negative aspiration, **hydrodissect** the fascial plane with sterile saline.
6. Once a homogeneous anechoic stripe is observed between the serratus and latissimus muscles, **inject** approximately 30 mL anesthetic.

Figure 1. Region of analgesia

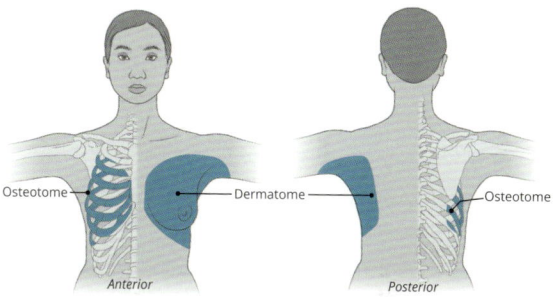

Osteotome — Dermatome — Osteotome

Anterior — Posterior

Figure 2 (below, left): Probe placement
Figure 3 (below, center and right): Ultrasound anatomy

1. Latissimus dorsi muscle
2. Serratus anterior muscle
3. Rib
4. Pleura

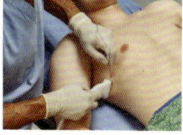
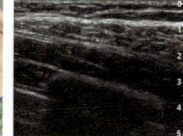
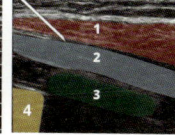

Pearls and Pitfalls

- Increasing volume (by dilution of LA), while staying within safe dose, can enhance spread and efficacy of block.
- Ensure you can visualize the lung in your field of view.
- Be aware of the thoracodorsal artery to avoid accidental puncture.
- Be careful performing this block in patients with chronic lung disease, given proximity to lung tissue.
- Debate exists between experts on increased risk of LAST from thoracic plane blocks. Several experts advocate for using lower than maximum doses.

ERECTOR SPINAE PLANE BLOCK

Materials *(adapt to patient, clinician, and site-specific factors/availability)*

Probe	High-frequency linear probe or curvilinear probe for more depth
Needle	80-100 mm, 22 G blunt tip needle Hyperechoic block needle with tubing
Volume of anesthetic	30-60 mL (dilute if needed; split dose between 2 syringes as needed)
Other	30-50 mL syringe, 10 mL sterile saline (for hydrodissection) Skin prep and PPE *Optional: 1-2 mL 1% lidocaine in separate syringe for skin wheal*

Region of Analgesia
Anesthetizes the posterior and lateral chest wall through complete blockade of the dorsal rami (and variable blockade of the ventral rami) that provide both visceral and somatic innervation. There is no motor involvement (**Figure 1**).

Indications	Contraindications
• Rib fractures • Thoracostomy insertion • Herpes zoster • Thoracic abscesses, burns, lacerations • Renal colic	• Overlying infection • Allergy to anesthetic • Anticoagulation (relative)

Patient Positioning
- Seated, facing away from the operator, with a pillow or table to lean on, similar to a lumbar puncture. Additionally, the patient can be in a lateral decubitus or prone position.

Procedure
1. Sterilize field per local guidelines.
2. With patient sitting upright, **place** probe over the midline thoracic spine in a sagittal orientation at midpoint of desired anesthesia on thoracic spine. Starting at the midline and moving laterally, **identify** the spinous process, lamina, flat transverse process, and rounded rib.
3. **Insert** needle in an in-line approach from the cephalad to caudal approach.
4. **Advance** under in-plane visualization such that the tip of the needle rests on the superficial aspect of the transverse process. After negative aspiration, **hydrodissect** the fascial plane with sterile saline to confirm placement.
5. Once confirmed, **inject** anesthetic, visualizing the spread of local anesthetic along the fascial plane.

Figure 1. Region of analgesia (with mid-thoracic injection)

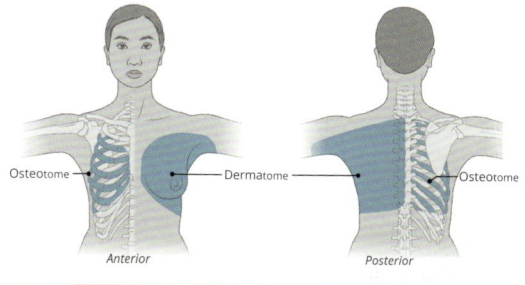

Anterior — Osteotome — Dermatome — Posterior — Osteotome

1. Trapezius 2. Rhomboid 3. Erector spinae 4. Transverse process 5. Pleura

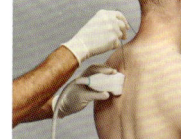 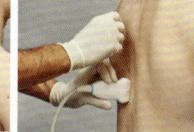 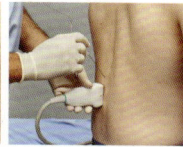

Figure 2 (above): Probe placement

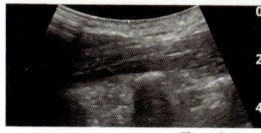 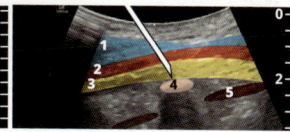

Figure 3 (above): Ultrasound anatomy

Pearls and Pitfalls

- Increasing volume (by diluting LA), while staying within safe dose, can enhance spread and efficacy. Avoid intramuscular injections by ensuring fascial spread.
- Use saline hydrodissection to aid in needle location and assure placement within the fascia.
- For single fractures or zoster, you can target the vertebra that correspond to the affected rib or dermatome.
- With multiple fractures, center the block such that cranial and caudal spread will maximize distribution to the affected dermatomes. Expect slightly more caudal than cranial spread.
- Debate exists between experts on increased risk of LAST from thoracic plane blocks. Several experts advocate for using lower than maximum doses.

TRANSVERSE ABDOMINUS PLANE (TAP) BLOCK

Materials *(adapt to patient, clinician, and site-specific factors/availability)*

Probe	High-frequency linear probe or curvilinear probe for more depth
Needle	50-100 mm, 22 G blunt tip needle Hyperechoic block needle with tubing
Volume of anesthetic	30-40 mL
Other	30-50 mL syringe, 10 mL sterile saline (for hydrodissection) Skin prep and PPE *Optional: 1-2 mL 1% lidocaine in separate syringe for skin wheal*

Region of Analgesia
Anesthetizes the lower abdominal wall, abdominal wall musculature, and parietal peritoneum through the anterior rami of spinal nerves (T7–L1), which includes intercostal nerves (T7–T11), the subcostal nerve, and the iliohypogastric and ilioinguinal nerves. The subcostal TAP block provides coverage from T6-T9 and the traditional/ lateral TAP block covers T10-T12 from the midline to the mid / posterior axillary line ranging from the umbilicus superiorly to the hypogastrium / upper thigh inferiorly. There is no motor involvement (**Figure 1**).

Indications	Contraindications
• Abdominal pain	• Allergy to local anesthetic
• Appendicitis	• Overlying infection
• Pre-operative pain relief for abdominal surgeries	• Anticoagulation (relative)
• Penetrating abdominal trauma requiring local wound exploration	• Cirrhosis (relative)
• Abdominal wall abscess, lacerations, burns	

Patient Positioning
- Supine and exposed from inferior costal margin to iliac crest

Procedure
1. Sterilize field per local guidelines.
2. **Place** probe transversely in midaxillary line at midpoint between iliac crest and inferior costal margin.
3. **Identify** subcutaneous tissue, external oblique muscle, internal oblique muscle, transverse abdominis muscle, and peritoneum.
4. Using an in-plane approach from medial to lateral, **advance** needle between internal oblique and transverse abdominis musculature.
5. After negative aspiration, **confirm** placement using hydrodissection to open the plane.
6. Once confirmed, **inject** full volume of anesthesia, watching spread through plane.

Figure 1. Region of analgesia

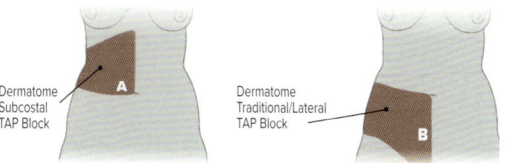

Dermatome Subcostal TAP Block

Dermatome Traditional/Lateral TAP Block

Figure 2 (photos below): Probe placement
  A. Subcostal TAP block
  B. Traditional/lateral TAP block

Figure 3 (US scans below): Ultrasound anatomy with lateral needle approach

1. External oblique
2. Internal oblique
3. Transversus abdominis
4. Peritoneal cavity

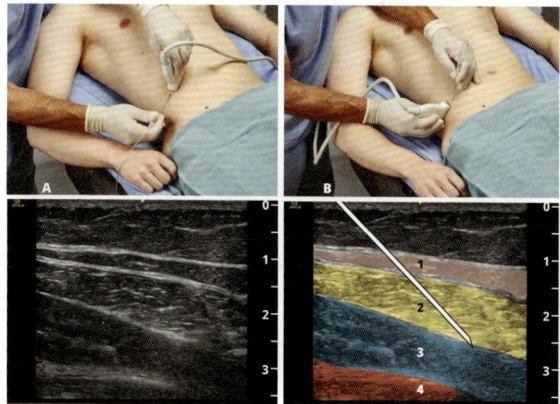

Pearls and Pitfalls

- Increasing volume (by dilution of LA), while staying within safe dose, can enhance spread and efficacy of block. Avoid intramuscular injections by ensuring fascial spread.
- Use a low angle of insertion, given this is a superficial block to avoid entering the peritoneal cavity and risking bowel injury.
- Consider for abdominal pain etiologies with somatic involvement; not as effective for visceral pain.

Upper Extremity

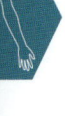

UPPER EXTREMITY

Interscalene Brachial Plexus Block 40

Supraclavicular Brachial Plexus Block 42

Suprascapular Nerve Block 44

Axillary Brachial Plexus Block 46

Ulnar Nerve Block 48

Radial Nerve Block 50

Median Nerve Block 52

Landmark-Based Hand Block 54

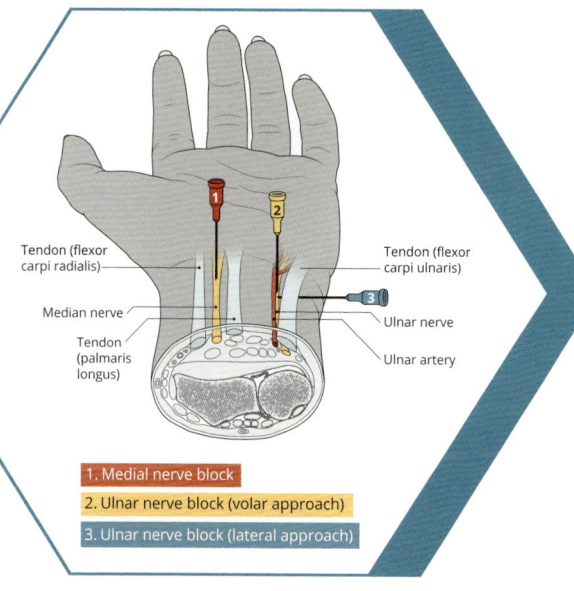

1. Medial nerve block
2. Ulnar nerve block (volar approach)
3. Ulnar nerve block (lateral approach)

INTERSCALENE BRACHIAL PLEXUS BLOCK

Materials *(adapt to patient, clinician, and site-specific factors/availability)*

Probe	High-frequency linear probe
Needle	50 mm, 22 G blunt tip needle Hyperechoic block needle with tubing
Volume of anesthetic	5-10 mL
Other	10 mL syringe, 10 mL sterile saline (for hydrodissection) Skin prep and PPE *Optional: 1-2 mL 1% lidocaine in separate syringe for skin wheal*

Region of Analgesia
Anesthetizes the shoulder and mid-humerus but does not reliably anesthetize the elbow and distal arm. Upper extremity motor paralysis can be expected for the duration of the block (**Figure 1**).

Indications	Contraindications
• Shoulder dislocations	• Allergy to local anesthetic
• Deltoid abscess for I&D	• Overlying infection
• Humeral head/neck/mid-shaft fractures	• Injuries at risk for compartment syndromes
• Distal clavicle fractures, burns, complex lacerations	• Anticoagulation (relative)
	• O_2 dependence or single lung on side of block (relative)

Patient Positioning
- Upright with head turned away from side of block. Alternatively, lateral decubitus with injured side up (**Figure 2**).

Procedure
1. Sterilize field per local guidelines.
2. **Place** linear transducer in supraclavicular fossa and identify pulsatile subclavian artery. Supraclavicular brachial plexus ("cluster of grapes") is lateral to artery.
3. **Slide** transducer cephalad, following brachial plexus into the interscalene groove where C5-7 nerve roots separate vertically, forming classic "traffic light." Note the interscalene brachial plexus is bordered medially by anterior scalene muscle and laterally by middle scalene muscle.
4. **Locate** target under prevertebral fascia overlying middle scalene muscle, 1-2 cm lateral to C5 nerve root. This fascial plane will allow spread of anesthetic into interscalene groove while avoiding risky interplexus injections.
5. Use in-plane approach to **advance** needle lateral-to-medial just under prevertebral fascia, superficial to middle scalene muscle.
6. After negative aspiration, use small aliquots of normal saline to **hydrodissect** fascial plane and look for spread into interscalene groove and around nerve roots of C5-7. Once satisfied with intrafascial spread, slowly **inject** additional 5-10 mL anesthetic to complete the block.

Figure 1. Region of analgesia

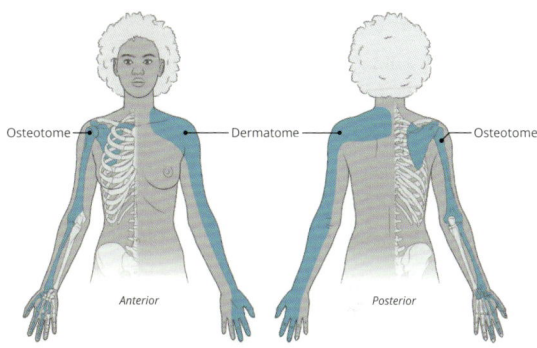

Anterior / Posterior

Figure 2 (left): Probe placement
Figure 3 (below): Ultrasound anatomy

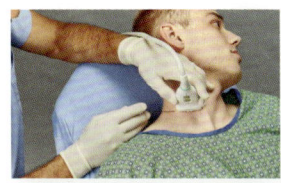

1. Sternocleidomastoid
2. Nerve roots
3. Anterior scalene
4. Middle scalene

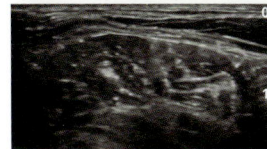
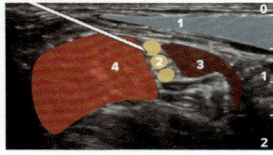

Pearls and Pitfalls

- Color Doppler can be used to identify and avoid vasculature.
- Spread of LA across and over C5/anterior scalene muscle indicates needle is superficial to prevertebral fascia and must be advanced 1-2 mm deeper.
- Larger volume increases the chance of phrenic nerve palsy (which occurs in 50% with 5 mL and 100% with 20 mL), but is well-tolerated by most patients.
- Be cautious if poor pulmonary function and/or contralateral pulmonary injury.
- To improve view, place a pillow or folded blanket behind affected shoulder.

SUPRACLAVICULAR BRACHIAL PLEXUS BLOCK

Materials *(adapt to patient, clinician, and site-specific factors/availability)*

Probe	High-frequency linear probe
Needle	50 mm, 22 G blunt tip needle
	Hyperechoic block needle with tubing
Volume of anesthetic	5-10 mL
Other	10 mL syringe, 10 mL sterile saline (for hydrodissection)
	Skin prep and PPE
	Optional: 1-2 mL 1% lidocaine in separate syringe for skin wheal

Region of Analgesia

The supraclavicular brachial plexus block is known as the "spinal of the arm," meaning it is generally the preferred block to provide analgesia to the entire arm. It typically results in motor paralysis from the mid-humerus distally for the duration of the block.
(Figure 1)

Indications	Contraindications
• Humeral fractures	• Allergy to local anesthetic
• Elbow fractures/dislocations	• Concern for forearm compartment syndrome
• Forearm lacerations/burns/abscesses	• Overlying infection
• Complex forearm/hand lacerations/burns	• Anticoagulation (relative)
• Hand injury/burn/infection	• O_2 dependence and/or single lung on side of block (relative contraindication

Patient Positioning

- Sitting upright or supine, with patient's head turned away from side of block (Figure 2)

Procedure

1. Sterilize field per local guidelines.
2. **Place** linear transducer parallel to clavicle into the supraclavicular fossa, posterior to mid-clavicle. **Identify** (in cross section) the pulsatile subclavian artery, which is lateral to carotid artery and superficial to first rib.
3. **Identify** supraclavicular brachial plexus that lies just lateral to subclavian artery, appearing as a hypoechoic "cluster of grapes."
4. Use color Doppler to **identify** any vascular structures and note the location of the sliding pleura on each side of the 1st rib.
5. Use an in-plane approach to carefully **advance** needle lateral-to-medial to the lateral border of brachial plexus, or until needle tip contacts first rib.
6. After negative aspiration, slowly **inject** while watching the anesthetic being deposited around or adjacent to nerve bundle.
7. **Redirect** needle as needed for anechoic circumferential spread of local anesthetic.

Figure 1. Region of analgesia

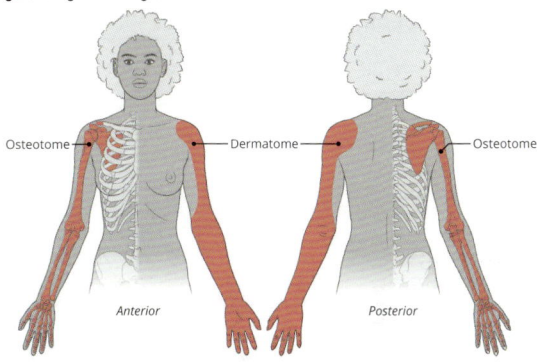

Osteotome — Dermatome — Osteotome

Anterior   Posterior

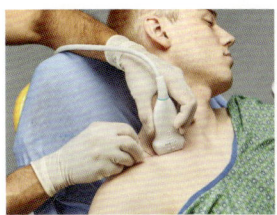

Figure 2 (left): Probe placement
Figure 3 (below): Ultrasound anatomy

1. Subclavian artery
2. Brachial plexus
3. First rib
4. Pleura

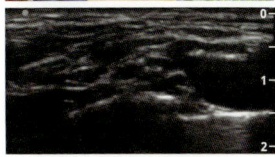
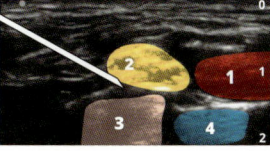

Pearls and Pitfalls

- If having difficulty identifying subclavian artery/brachial plexus complex, follow carotid artery in neck caudally into supraclavicular fossa, then slide laterally.
- Larger-volume blocks may provide anesthesia to the shoulder.
- Be cautious in patients with pulmonary disease (60% incidence of phrenic nerve paralysis with 25 mL anesthetic).

SUPRASCAPULAR NERVE BLOCK

Materials *(adapt to patient, clinician, and site-specific factors/availability)*

Probe	High-frequency linear probe
Needle	80-100 mm, 22 G blunt tip needle Hyperechoic block needle with tubing
Volume of anesthetic	10-15 mL
Other	10-20 mL syringe, 10 mL sterile saline (for hydrodissection) Skin prep and PPE *Optional: 1-2 mL 1% lidocaine in separate syringe for skin wheal*

Region of Analgesia

Anesthetizes the scapula as well as the shoulder joint through its innervation of the C5 nerve root. It is expected there will be motor dysfunction to the supraspinatus and infraspinatus muscles (**Figure 1**).

Indications	Contraindications
• Scapular fractures • Acute or chronic shoulder pain	• Allergy to local anesthetic • Overlying infection • Anticoagulation (relative)

Patient Positioning
- Upright with head turned away from side of the block. Alternatively, lateral decubitus with injured side up (**Figure 2**).

Procedure
1. Sterilize field per local guidelines.
2. **Locate** spine of scapula and place probe transversely, cephalad to scapular spine, "down" into scapular fossa.
3. **Identify** suprascapular notch below supraspinatus muscle. The notch can be seen as a "break" in the bony line of the supraspinatus fossa. The superior transverse scapular ligament overlies the notch. Pulsation of the suprascapular artery may be visible.
4. Using in-plane approach from lateral to medial, **direct** the needle to transverse the trapezius and supraspinatus muscle until needle tip is above the superior transverse scapular ligament.
5. After negative aspiration, **hydrodissect** fascial plane with sterile saline.
6. Once confirmed, **inject** approximately 10-15 mL anesthetic.

Figure 1. Region of analgesia

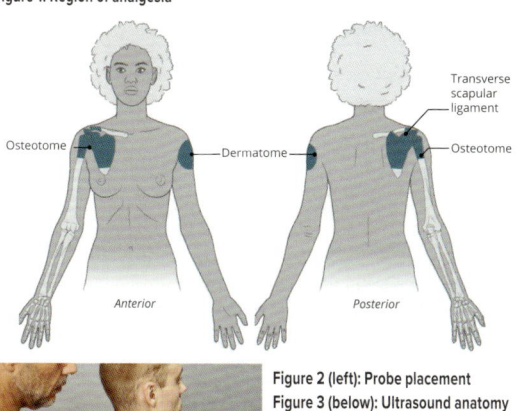

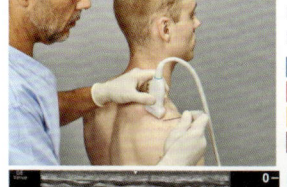

Figure 2 (left): Probe placement
Figure 3 (below): Ultrasound anatomy

1. Trapezius
2. Supraspinatus
3. Suprascapular nerve
4. Suprascapular notch outline

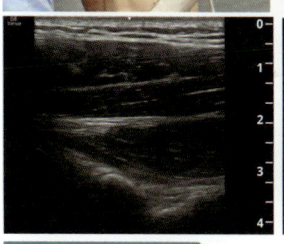
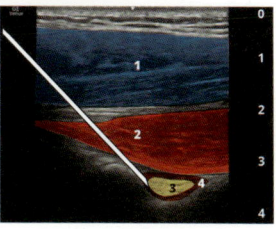

Pearls and Pitfalls

- Ultrasound visualization may improve when patient places affected hand on unaffected shoulder.
- Avoid entering the suprascapular notch, as there is risk of causing a pneumothorax. Excessive needle movement anteriorly through the notch can result in pleural puncture.

AXILLARY BRACHIAL PLEXUS BLOCK

Materials *(adapt to patient, clinician, and site-specific factors/availability)*

Probe	High-frequency linear probe
Needle	50 mm, 22 G blunt tip needle Hyperechoic block needle with tubing
Volume of anesthetic	20-40 mL
Other	20-50 mL syringe Skin prep and PPE *Optional: 1-2 mL 1% lidocaine in separate syringe for skin wheal*

Region of Analgesia
This block involves the arm below the shoulder and axilla level; it does not block the axilla or shoulder but does affect motor function (**Figure 1**).

Indications	Contraindications
• Colles fracture, hand/wrist/forearm/elbow laceration • Burns • Pain below mid-humeral level	• Allergy to local anesthetic • Overlying infection • Injuries with high risk of compartment syndrome (forearm fractures, supracondylar fractures)

Patient Positioning
- Supine, arm raised, hand under the occiput (**Figure 2**)

Procedure
1. **Place** transducer in transverse plane, relative to axillary artery at anterior edge of axilla.
2. **Identify** median, radial, and ulnar nerves adjacent to artery, then identify musculocutaneous nerve between biceps and coracobrachialis muscles.
3. **Inject** 20-40 mL deep to the axillary artery.

Pearls and Pitfalls
- A single perivascular injection works as well as multiple injections adjacent to median, radial, and ulnar nerves.
- This block can be performed more distal in the region of the proximal one-third of the upper arm as well.

Figure 1. Region of analgesia

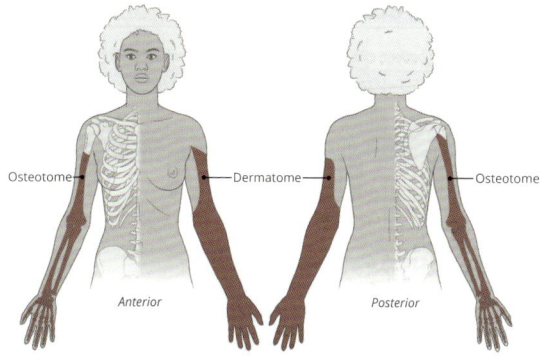

Anterior   Posterior

Figure 2 (left): Probe placement
Figure 3 (below): Ultrasound anatomy

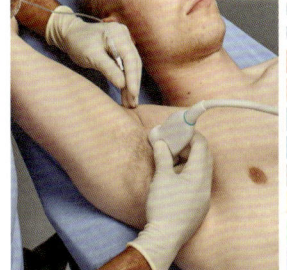

1. Axillary artery
2. Axillary vein
3. Radial nerve
4. Median nerve
5. Ulnar nerve
6. Musculocutaneous nerve
7. Biceps brachialis muscle
8. Coracobrachialis muscle

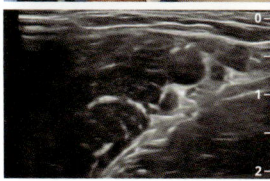
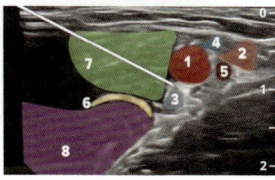

Upper Extremity

2023 EMRA and AAED Nerve Block Guide

RADIAL NERVE BLOCK

Materials *(adapt to patient, clinician, and site-specific factors/availability)*

Probe	High-frequency linear probe
Needle	50 mm, 22 G blunt tip needle
	Hyperechoic block needle preferred, tubing optional
Volume of anesthetic	5-10 mL
Other	10 mL syringe
	Skin prep and PPE
	Optional: 1-2 mL 1% lidocaine in separate syringe for skin wheal

Region of Analgesia
Anesthetizes the radial aspect of the hand on the dorsum, as well as the dorsum of the first three and a half fingers. This block may lead to a wrist drop (**Figure 1**).

Indications	Contraindications
• Fracture and dislocation of lateral aspect of forearm and hand	• Allergy to local anesthetic
• Laceration and abscesses to posterior aspect of forearm and radial aspect of the dorsum of hand	• Overlying infection
• Post-op and pre-op anesthesia	• Anticoagulation (relative)
• Burns, tendon repairs	

Patient Positioning
- Supine or sitting up in bed with ipsilateral arm bent at elbow, shoulder internally rotated. Arm may be resting on bedside table or on chest/abdomen (**Figure 2**).

Procedure
1. Sterilize field per local guidelines.
2. **Place** probe in transverse orientation over anterolateral aspect of distal humerus, about 4 cm proximal (superior) to lateral epicondyle.
3. Nerve will be visualized as a **hyperechoic triangular structure** within a fascial plane between the brachialis (inferior) and brachioradialis (superior) muscles.
4. **Place** transducer transversely and use an in-plane needle approach from either side, depending on the ergonomic needs of the operator, so needle tip lies superior or inferior to radial nerve.
5. Once satisfied, **aspirate** and then **inject** 1 mL anesthetic to evaluate placement by watching the anesthetic spread.
6. Once confirmed, **inject** remaining anesthetic.

Figure 1. Region of analgesia

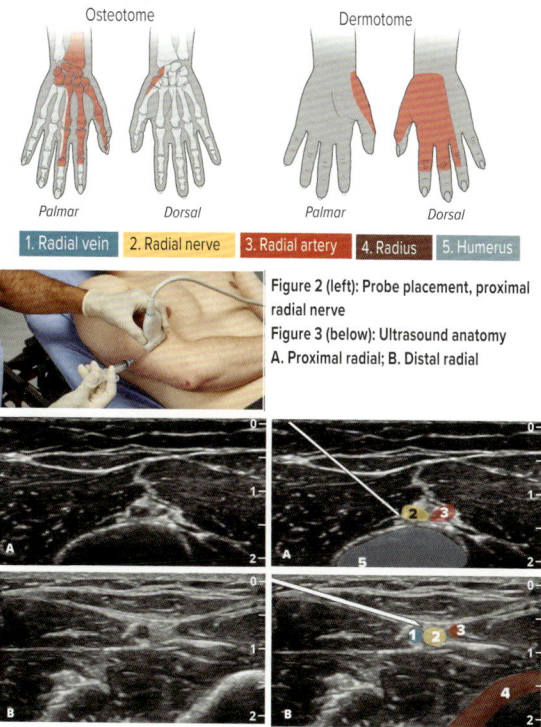

Figure 2 (left): Probe placement, proximal radial nerve
Figure 3 (below): Ultrasound anatomy
A. Proximal radial; B. Distal radial

Upper Extremity

Pearls and Pitfalls

- Perform with ulnar and/or medial nerve blocks for a complete hand block.
- To avoid motor blockade, block distal to the elbow crease, past the point of bifurcation, into superficial sensory and deep motor branches.
- Circumferential spread of LA around nerve is not necessary for this block. A pool of LA immediately adjacent to either the posterolateral or anterior aspect is sufficient.

MEDIAN NERVE BLOCK

Materials *(adapt to patient, clinician, and site-specific factors/availability)*

Probe	High-frequency linear probe
Needle	50 mm, 22 G blunt tip needle Hyperechoic block needle preferred, tubing optional
Volume of anesthetic	5-10 mL
Other	10 mL syringe Skin prep and PPE

Region of Analgesia
Anesthetizes the radial aspect of the palm, and the palmar aspect and respective nail bed of the index and middle fingers, part of the thumb and part of the ring finger (some sensory innervation variability of the fingers). This block may affect flexion of the first three fingers and thumb opposition, resulting in the benediction sign when trying to make a fist (**Figure 1**).

Indications	Contraindications
• Abscess drainage or laceration repair in the median nerve distribution (eg palmar) • Pain control for burns, large abrasions and avulsions for debridement • Fracture or dislocation to the hand (consider combining with ulnar and radial nerve blocks)	• Allergy to local anesthetic • Overlying infection • Concern for compartment syndrome • Anticoagulation (relative)

Patient Positioning
- Seated or semi-recumbent. Support/rest forearm to side of patient on pillow or table, with hand in supination. Place US machine across from operator for best visualization (**Figure 2**).

Procedure
1. **Place** linear probe in transverse plane with marker to operator's left on the volar surface of the mid-forearm. The median nerve will be the hyperechoic bundle in the plane between the flexor digitorum superficialis and flexor digitorum profundus, in the midline of the forearm.
2. **Target injection** to facial plane, surrounding the nerve with 5-10 mL of anesthetic. Use an in-plane technique for continuous needle visualization.

Figure 1. Region of analgesia

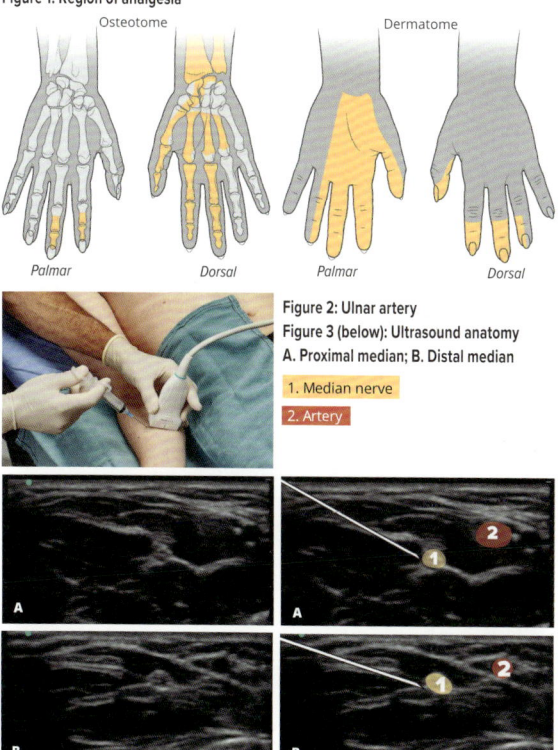

Osteotome — Palmar, Dorsal
Dermatome — Palmar, Dorsal

Figure 2: Ulnar artery
Figure 3 (below): Ultrasound anatomy
A. Proximal median; B. Distal median

1. Median nerve
2. Artery

Upper Extremity

Pearls and Pitfalls

- Good visualization of nerves is important — using a nerve preset and understanding the concept of anisotropy (angle generated artifact) will help.
- The median nerve is more easily distinguished in the mid-forearm.
- The ulnar aspect of the palm is not covered by the median nerve, so an ulnar and/or radial nerve block may also be necessary to achieve a total block.

LANDMARK-BASED HAND BLOCK

Materials *(adapt to patient, clinician, and site-specific factors/availability)*

Needle	25 G, 1.5" blunt tip needle
Volume of anesthetic	10-15 mL
Other	10-20 mL syringe
	Skin prep and PPE
	Optional: 1-2 mL 1% lidocaine in separate syringe for skin wheal

Region of Analgesia
The hand is innervated by the median, ulnar, and radial nerves. The ulnar nerve provides sensation to the skin on the entire fifth digit, half of the fourth digit, and the ulnar aspect of the hand and wrist. The median nerve innervates the skin of the lateral 3.5 fingers, except the dorsal aspect of the thumb and the corresponding area of the palm. The radial nerve provides sensory innervation to the dorsal lateral half of the hand and the dorsal aspect of the thumb. The digital nerves branch off the median and ulnar nerves in the distal palm and travel on either side of the flexor tendon sheath, innervating the respective finger (**Figure 1**). [For specific motor involvement, refer to p. 48-52.]

Indications	Contraindications
• Fracture/dislocation reduction of respective osteotome being blocked	• Allergy to local anesthetic
• Abscess drainage or laceration repair	• Overlying infection
• Burns	• Concern for compartment syndrome
	• Anticoagulation (relative)

Patient Positioning
■ Supine, semi-recumbent, or upright with arm abducted and hand resting on a procedure table/flat surface

Procedure
Sterilize field per local guidelines, then refer to specific procedures listed on following pages. Consider optional skin wheal as preferred.

Figure 1. Region of analgesia

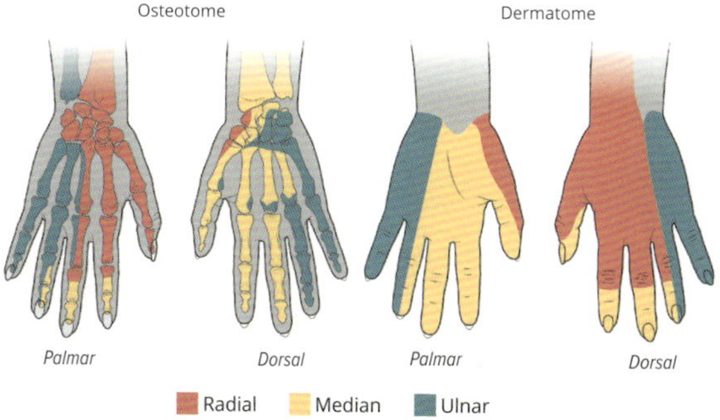

Osteotome — Palmar, Dorsal
Dermatome — Palmar, Dorsal

- Radial
- Median
- Ulnar

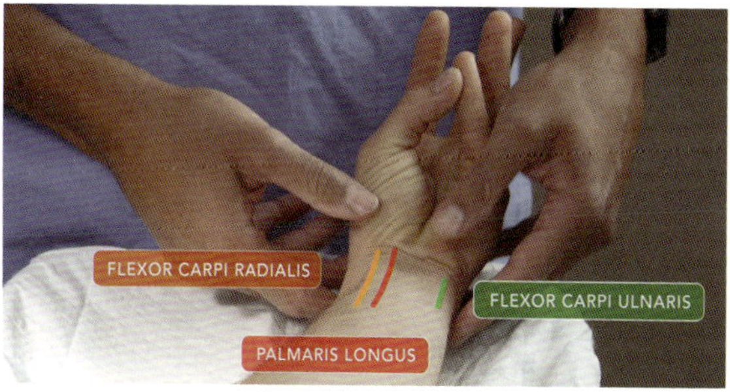

Figure 2: Anatomic landmarks (FLEXOR CARPI RADIALIS, PALMARIS LONGUS, FLEXOR CARPI ULNARIS)

Pearls and Pitfalls

- Good visualization of the nerves is important — using a nerve preset and understanding the concept of anisotropy (angle generated artifact) will help improve nerve visualization.
- Median nerve is more easily located in the mid-forearm, as closer to the wrist it can be difficult to distinguish from surrounding tendons.
- The ulnar aspect of the palm is not covered by the median nerve, so some injuries may require an ulnar and/or radial nerve block in addition to a median nerve block.

Ulnar nerve block

1. Recommend lateral (ulnar) approach because volar approach has been associated with increased risk of vascular injury or injection.
2. With the palm facing up, **identify** the injection site, which is 1-2 cm proximal to the wrist crease and on the ulnar aspect of the wrist, immediately deep to the flexor carpi ulnaris.
3. **Advance** the needle under the flexor carpi ulnaris, approximately 0.5-1 cm towards the radial side of the wrist.
4. **Aspirate** to rule out vascular placement, and **inject** approximately 5 mL of anesthetic. If blood is aspirated, withdraw the needle a few mm, as the nerve is ulnar to the artery.
5. Consider an additional block of the cutaneous branches of the ulnar nerve: **inject** 3-5 mL of LA just superficial to the flexor carpi ulnaris.

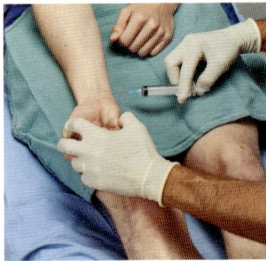
Figure 3: Needle placement, ulnar nerve block

Median nerve block

1. With palm facing up, **identify** injection site just lateral (radial) to palmaris longus and medial to flexor carpi radialis, at the proximal wrist crease.
2. **Advance** the needle perpendicular to the skin until it pierces the deep fascia. If fascial "pop" is not felt, advance until needle hits bone and withdraw 2-5 mm, then **inject** 5 mL of anesthetic.
3. **Withdraw** needle and **reinsert** both 30° medially and 30° laterally, injecting additional 2-3 mL anesthetic on each side to improve efficacy.

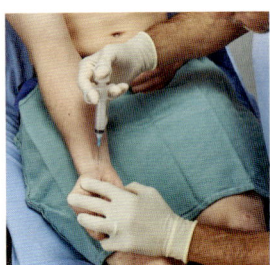
Figure 4: Needle placement, median nerve block

Radial nerve block

1. With palm facing down and thumb up, **locate** radial styloid and anatomic snuff box. **Identify** the injection site at the radial styloid.
2. **Inject** a total of 5-7 mL of anesthetic just above radial styloid, extending both medially and laterally. The superficial branch of the radial nerve crosses above the radial styloid and branches to the dorsum of the thumb, index finger, and lateral half of the middle finger. Due to significant anatomic variability, consider the radial nerve block to be a field block that bathes the distribution of the radial nerve in anesthetic.

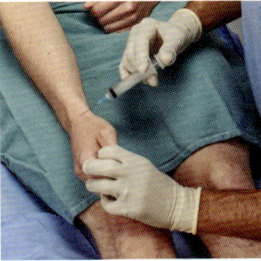

Figure 5: Needle placement, radial nerve block

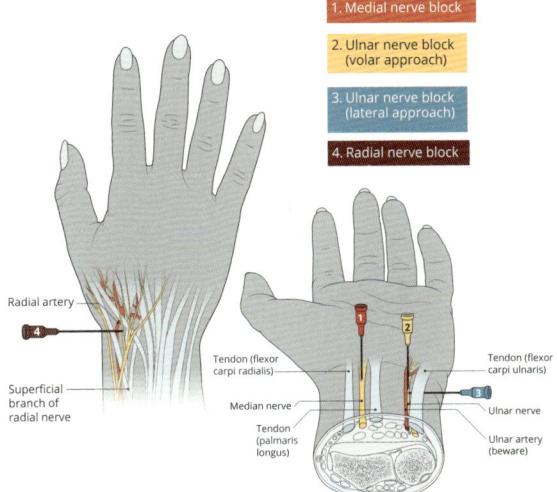

Figure 6: Needle placement

Upper Extremity

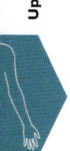

LOWER EXTREMITY

PENG Block 60

Transgluteal Sciatic Nerve Block 62

Infrainguinal Fascia Iliaca Plane Block 64

Saphenous Nerve / Adductor Canal Block 66

Distal Sciatic Nerve Block in Popliteal Fossa 68

Ankle Block 70

Distal Tibial Nerve Block 72

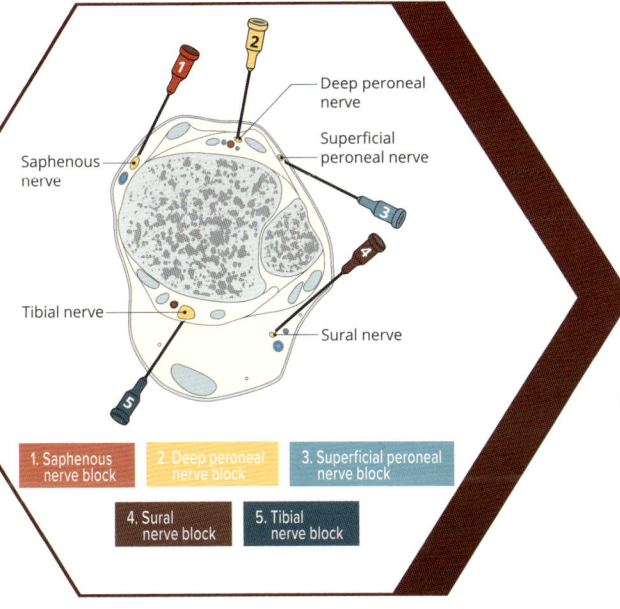

PERISCAPULAR NERVE GROUP (PENG) BLOCK

Materials *(adapt to patient, clinician, and site-specific factors/availability)*

Probe	Curvilinear probe
Needle	80-100 mm, 22 G blunt tip block needle
	Hyperechoic block needle with tubing
Volume of anesthetic	20-30 mL
Other	30 mL syringe; 10 mL sterile saline (for hydrodissection)
	Skin prep and PPE
	Optional: 1-2 mL 1% lidocaine in separate syringe for skin wheal

Region of Analgesia

May provide more complete anesthesia for hip fractures compared to femoral or fascia iliaca blocks. It anesthetizes the femoral head, neck, acetabulum, and pubic rami through the sensory nerves of the anterior capsule of the hip joint. The benefit of the PENG is anesthesia of the acetabulum and pubic rami; there is no motor involvement. **(Figure 1)**.

Indications	Contraindications
• Acetabular fractures	• Allergy to local anesthetic
• Pubic rami fractures	• Overlying infection
• Femoral neck fractures	• Anticoagulation (relative)
• Intertrochanteric fractures	

Patient Positioning
- Supine, leg externally rotated with the inguinal area exposed

Procedure
1. Sterilize field per local guidelines.
2. **Place** curvilinear probe at an oblique angle parallel and just inferior to the inguinal ligament to identify the femoral head and the femoral artery medially.
3. Move probe cranially to **identify** the anterior inferior iliac spine (AIIS) and the iliopubic rami. In this view, the femoral artery, femoral nerve, iliacus muscle, and psoas tendon should be seen. Target is the subfascial plane underneath the psoas tendon, above the ilium.
4. **Insert** blunt tip needle using in-plane orientation until tip is positioned between the psoas tendon and bone, avoiding femoral vessels and nerve.
5. After negative aspiration, **confirm** placement with hydrodissection to open planes, then **relax** probe pressure to allow easier injection.
6. Once confirmed, **inject** 20-30 mL anesthetic, visualizing the spread along the ilium elevating the iliacus muscle off the bone.

Figure 1. Region of analgesia

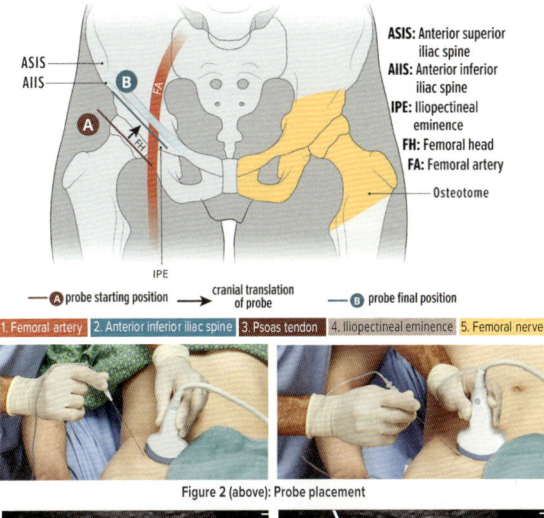

ASIS: Anterior superior iliac spine
AIIS: Anterior inferior iliac spine
IPE: Iliopectineal eminence
FH: Femoral head
FA: Femoral artery

— A probe starting position → cranial translation of probe — B probe final position

1. Femoral artery 2. Anterior inferior iliac spine 3. Psoas tendon 4. Iliopectineal eminence 5. Femoral nerve

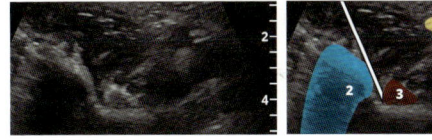

Figure 2 (above): Probe placement

Figure 3 (above): Ultrasound anatomy

Pearls and Pitfalls

- Bone can be more easily visualized in elderly patients with atrophied muscle and fascial layers that can make plane blocks difficult.
- This is a newer block similar to the fascia iliaca and femoral blocks; it anesthetizes the articular branches of the femoral, obturator, and accessory obturator nerves.
- Intramuscular injection in the iliacus may result in anesthesia of the femoral nerve, resulting in quadriceps weakness.
- Pelvic fractures may result in hematoma formation along the ilium. Aspiration of blood at the ilium should prompt repositioning of the needle. If still aspirating blood, the procedure should be aborted.

TRANSGLUTEAL SCIATIC NERVE BLOCK

Materials *(adapt to patient, clinician, and site-specific factors/availability)*

Probe	Curvilinear probe (or high-frequency probe for shallower depth)
Needle	100-120 mm, 22 G blunt tip needle
	Hyperechoic block needle with tubing
Volume of anesthetic	10-20 mL
Other	20-30 mL syringe; 10 mL sterile saline (for hydrodissection)
	Skin prep and PPE
	Optional: 1-2 mL 1% lidocaine in separate syringe for skin wheal

Region of Analgesia
Anesthetizes the posterior upper leg, knee distal to the site of the block, below-the-knee sensation except to the medial malleolus, and medial leg including the hamstring muscles. There is potential to develop a transient foot drop from this block (**Figure 1**).

Indications	Contraindications
• Acute or acute-on-chronic sciatica	• Allergy to local anesthetic
• Lower leg/ankle fracture/dislocation	• Overlying infection
• Lower extremity lacerations/burns/abscesses	• Concern for compartment syndrome
	• Anticoagulation (relative)

Patient Positioning
- Lateral decubitus position, with affected extremity facing up so hips and knees are flexed to patient's comfort

Procedure
1. Sterilize field per local guidelines.
2. **Place** probe in transverse orientation on posterior buttocks between greater trochanter of the femur and ischial tuberosity.
3. **Identify** sciatic nerve as triangular structure deep to gluteal maximus fascial layer, between bony landmarks of greater trochanter of femur and the ischial tuberosity. Target is immediately adjacent to sciatic nerve under gluteal maximus muscle.
4. **Insert** needle either laterally or medially, using in-plane approach to guide needle under the gluteal maximus fascial layer. A high angle approach is advised.
5. After negative aspiration, **confirm** needle placement using hydrodissection to open the plane. Once confirmed, **inject** 10-20 mL anesthetic.

Pearls and Pitfalls
- An infragluteal approach, with probe placed transverse along the gluteal crease, may be used if structures are better visualized.

Figure 1. Region of analgesia

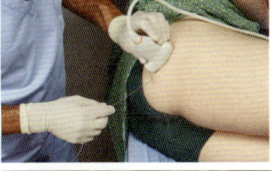
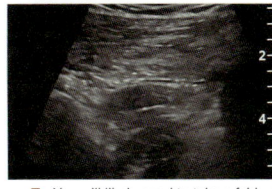

Osteotome — Dermatome — Osteotome

Anterior *Posterior*

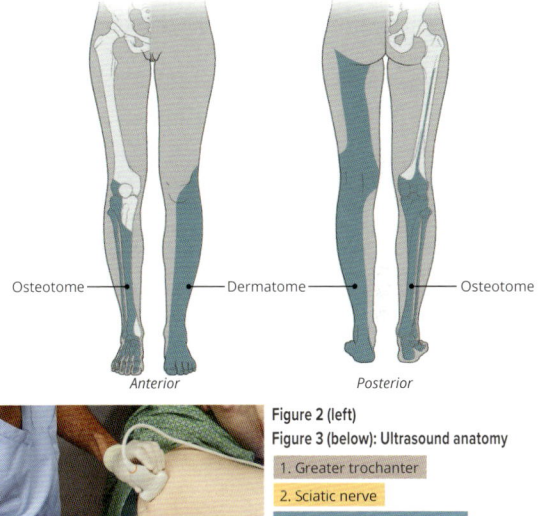

Figure 2 (left)
Figure 3 (below): Ultrasound anatomy

1. Greater trochanter
2. Sciatic nerve
3. Gluteus maximus muscle
4. Ischial tuberosity
5. Quadratus femoris muscle

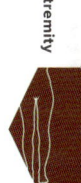

Lower Extremity

- You will likely need to take a fairly steep angle of approach to reach the injection target, given the relative depth of the sciatic nerve.
- The sciatic nerve is large; repeated needle repositioning and anesthetic injections may be needed to deliver anesthetic circumferentially.

INFRAINGUINAL FASCIA ILIACA PLANE BLOCK

Materials *(adapt to patient, clinician, and site-specific factors/availability)*

Probe	High-frequency linear probe
Needle	80-100 mm, 22 G blunt tip needle
	Hyperechoic block needle with tubing
Volume of anesthetic	30-40 mL
Other	50 mL syringe; 10 mL sterile saline (for hydrodissection)
	Skin prep and PPE
	Optional: 1-2 mL 1% lidocaine in separate syringe for skin wheal

Region of Analgesia
Anesthetizes the anterior and medial thigh, hip joint, knee, and medial side of the leg from the knee to the foot. This block may cause weakness in knee extension, abduction, and flexion (**Figure 1**).

Indications	Contraindications
• Hip fracture	• Allergy to local anesthetic
• Femur fracture	• Overlying infection
• Anterior thigh lacerations/abscesses	• Anticoagulation (relative)

Patient Positioning
- Supine, groin exposed to identify anterior superior iliac spine and inguinal crease

Procedure
1. Sterilize field per local guidelines.
2. **Place** probe parallel and just below inguinal crease to visualize the femoral artery and femoral nerve as well as overlying fascia iliaca.
3. **Advance** with in-plane visualization, using a lateral-to-medial visual approach so blunt needle tip lies lateral to femoral nerve.
4. After negative aspiration, **hydrodissect** the fascial plane with sterile saline to confirm placement. Anechoic fluid should travel medially toward femoral artery but should not track superficially to artery.
5. Once confirmed, **inject** ~30 mL anesthetic, visualizing spread of LA along fascial plane.

Pearls and Pitfalls
- Increasing volume (by dilution of LA), while staying within safe dose, can enhance spread and efficacy of block. Avoid intramuscular injections by ensuring fascial spread.
- If probe is too distal, femoral artery will bifurcate and anatomy will be distorted.
- Ensure needle is not directed at femoral nerve, but rather aim lateral so fluid can be placed under the fascia iliaca.
- Ensure probe is parallel to inguinal ligament to see femoral artery in cross-section.

Figure 1. Region of analgesia

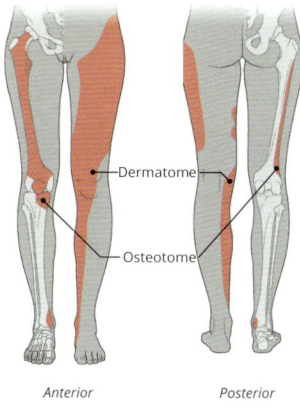

Dermatome
Osteotome

Anterior *Posterior*

Figure 2 (photo, right): Probe placement

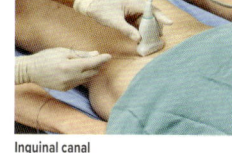

Inguinal canal

1. Fascia Lata 2. Fascia Iliaca 3. Femoral artery 4. Femoral nerve 5. Iliopsoas muscle
6. Sartorius

Figure 3 (below): Ultrasound anatomy
A. Infrainguinal fascia iliaca plane block; B. Femoral nerve block

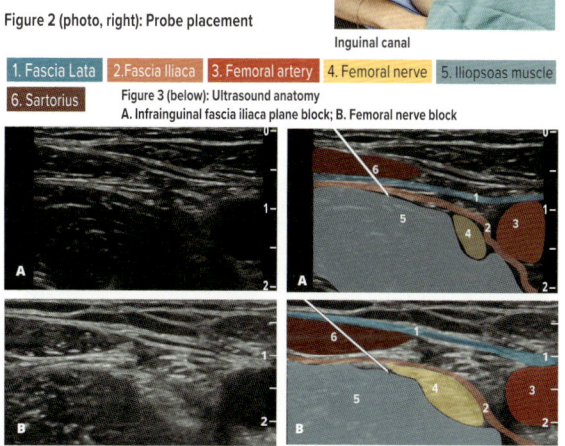

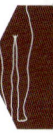

Lower Extremity

SAPHENOUS NERVE / ADDUCTOR CANAL BLOCK

Materials *(adapt to patient, clinician, and site-specific factors/availability)*

Probe	High-frequency linear probe
Needle	80-100 mm, 22 G blunt tip needle
	Hyperechoic block needle with tubing
Volume of anesthetic	20-30 mL
Other	20-30 mL syringe; 10 mL sterile saline (for hydrodissection)
	Skin prep and PPE
	Optional: 1-2 mL 1% lidocaine in separate syringe for skin wheal

Region of Analgesia
Anesthetizes the medial aspect of the lower leg and ankle as well as the anterior knee joint, including the patella. This block may cause mild quadriceps weakness, but much less than the femoral nerve block (**Figure 1**).

Indications	Contraindications
• Ligamentous knee injury	• Allergy to local anesthetic
• Patellar fracture/dislocation	• Overlying infection
• Ankle fracture/dislocation (when combined with popliteal sciatic block or proximal sciatic block)	• Anticoagulation (relative)

Patient Positioning
- Supine, with affected leg externally rotated at hip (ie, frog-leg position)

Procedure
1. Sterilize field per local guidelines.
2. **Place** transducer transversely on medial portion of thigh, at level of mid-femur.
3. **Identify** superficial femoral artery first, then find saphenous nerve adjacent to artery. The sartorius muscle is visualized on top of the artery and is the "roof" of the adductor canal.
4. Using an in-plane approach, **direct** the needle through sartorius muscle toward artery. Direct needle through posterior fascia of sartorius muscle. Target is through fascia at lower edge of sartorius muscle, adjacent to artery.
5. After negative aspiration, **hydrodissect** the fascial plane with sterile saline.
6. Once confirmed, **inject** 20–30 mL anesthetic around nerve and other structures.

Pearls and Pitfalls
- It is OK to perform more proximal in the leg, but you may risk more quadriceps weakness.
- Saphenous nerve may be difficult to appreciate prior to injection, and will be easier to visualize with hydrodissection.

Figure 1. Region of analgesia

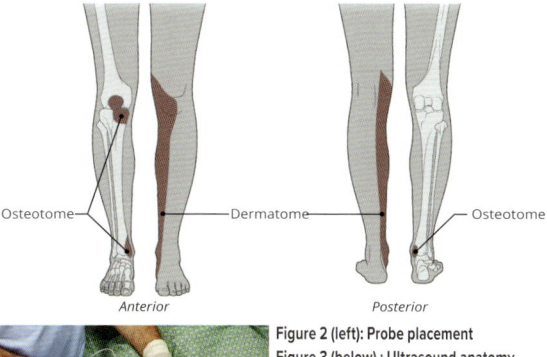

Anterior — Posterior

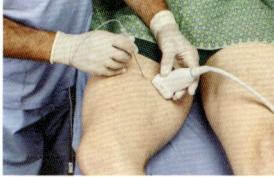

Figure 2 (left): Probe placement
Figure 3 (below): Ultrasound anatomy

1. Femoral vein
2. Saphenous nerve
3. Femoral artery
4. Sartorius
5. Vastus medialis muscle
6. Adductor longus/magnus

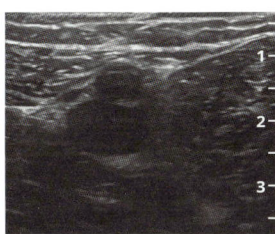
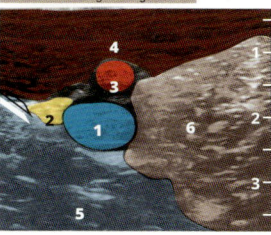

Lower Extremity

- The vein is often not visualized because it is relatively easily compressed by any pressure from the transducer.
- Avoid intramuscular injection into sartorius muscle or block will not have intended outcome.

DISTAL SCIATIC NERVE BLOCK IN POPLITEAL FOSSA

Materials *(adapt to patient, clinician, and site-specific factors/availability)*

Probe	High-frequency linear probe
Needle	50-100 mm, 22 G blunt tip needle
	Hyperechoic block needle with tubing
Volume of anesthetic	20-30 mL
Other	20-30 mL syringe; 10 mL sterile saline (for hydrodissection)
	Skin prep and PPE
	Optional: 1-2 mL 1% lidocaine in separate syringe for skin wheal

Region of Analgesia
Anesthetizes the lower leg, except medial malleolus and medial leg. This block allows for knee flexion but causes weakness of muscles distal to the knee joint (**Figure 1**).

Indications	Contraindications
• Ankle fracture/dislocation (best when combined with saphenous nerve block)	• Allergy to local anesthetic
• Lower extremity lacerations/burns/abscesses	• Overlying infection
• Calcaneus fractures, Achilles tendon rupture	• Concern for compartment syndrome
	• Anticoagulation (relative)

Patient Positioning
- Prone, allowing easy access to popliteal fossa. If patient is unable to lie prone, elevate and support the affected extremity, with mild flexion of the knee.

Procedure
1. Sterilize field per local guidelines.
2. **Place** linear probes transversely, just proximal to popliteal crease, and identify the "snowman" of the tibial nerve, popliteal vein, and artery.
3. Scan cranially to **identify** bifurcation of sciatic nerve into tibial and common peroneal nerves that lies ~5-10 cm proximal to the popliteal crease. Target will be immediately distal to bifurcation of sciatic nerve since they share a common sheath.
4. **Insert** needle lateral to medial, using in-plane visualization with probe at the level of the bifurcation, until needle tip is between tibial and common peroneal nerves.
5. After negative aspiration, **confirm** needle placement using hydrodissection to open the planes. Once confirmed, **inject** 20-30 mL anesthetic.

Pearls and Pitfalls
- Avoid in patients with mid-tibial fractures to avoid masking compartment syndrome.
- Below the knee this block only spares the medial leg/malleolus.
- Combine with the adductor canal block to give complete anesthesia below the knee. This is especially useful for reduction of ankle fractures and dislocations.
- Often called a popliteal nerve block, although there is no popliteal nerve.

Figure 1. Region of analgesia

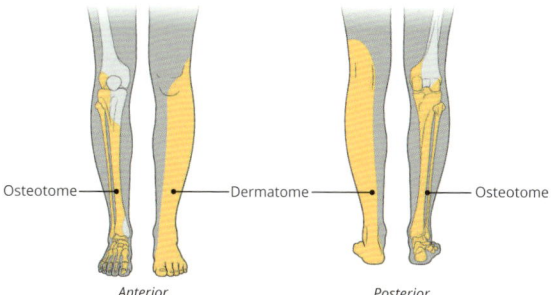

Anterior — Osteotome, Dermatome
Posterior — Osteotome

Figure 2 (below): Probe placement

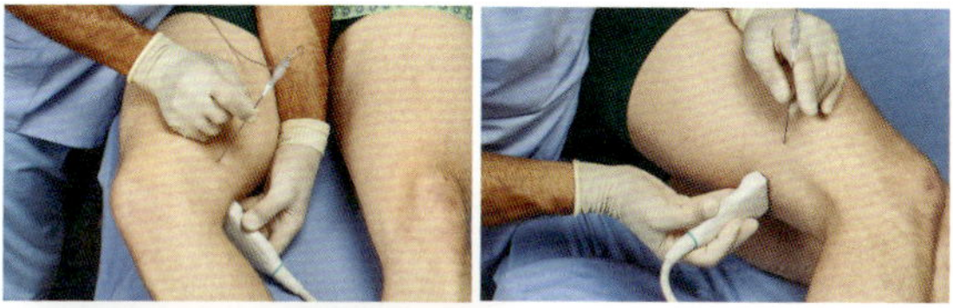

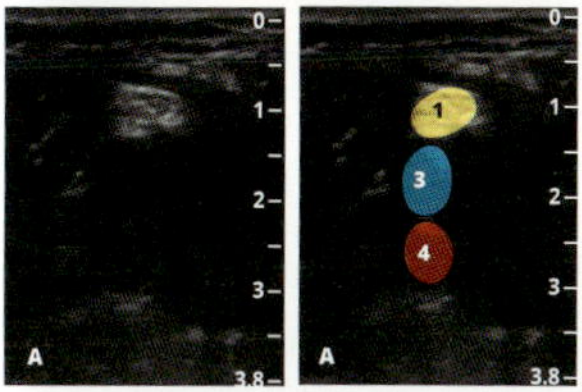

Figure 3 (left, below): Ultrasound anatomy
A. At popliteal crease;
B. At the bifurcation of the sciatic nerve

1. Tibial nerve
2. Sciatic nerve bifurcating to tibial and common peroneal nerves
3. Popliteal vein
4. Popliteal artery

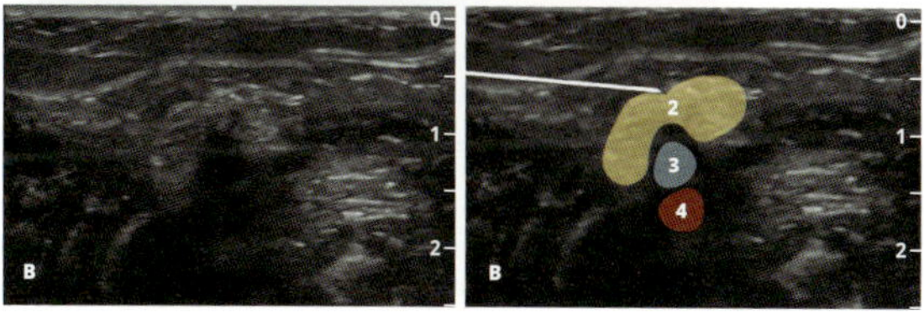

Lower Extremity

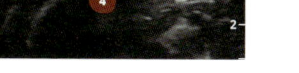

ANKLE BLOCK

Materials *(adapt to patient, clinician, and site-specific factors/availability)*

Probe	High-frequency linear probe
Needle	50 mm, 25 G blunt tip needle; tubing optional
Volume of anesthetic	10-15 mL
Other	10-20 mL syringe Skin prep and PPE

Region of Analgesia

Saphenous nerve: Afferent branch of femoral nerve; innervates instep of foot and medial ankle. Can be used in isolation for lacerations, or in addition to sciatic block for ankle fracture/dislocation.
Deep peroneal nerve: Innervates webspace between 1st and 2nd toes on dorsum of foot.
Superficial peroneal nerve: Innervates most of the dorsum of foot.
Sural nerve: Innervates posterolateral calf and dorsolateral foot.
Distal tibial nerve: Covers sensation on heel and sole, except a small region of the instep and a sliver of skin on lateral surface of the sole. Consider for foreign body removal, laceration to sole, or calcaneal fracture.

Indications	Contraindications
• Lacerations • Abscesses/foreign body removal • Fractures/dislocations involving affected dermatome or osteotome	• Allergy to local anesthetic • Overlying infection • Concern for compartment syndrome • Anticoagulation (relative)

Patient Positioning and Procedure

Sterilize field per local guidelines.

Saphenous nerve block (mid-thigh or below knee)
- **Position** supine with leg abducted and externally rotated (ie, frogleg) to allow access to medial thigh
- **Place** probe proximal to medial malleolus and identify saphenous nerve anteriorly to saphenous vein.
- **Inject** 3-5 mL local anesthetic.

Deep peroneal nerve block
- **Position** supine to access anterior ankle.
- **Place** probe transverse along anterolateral aspect of lower leg, proximal to ankle. Nerve lies lateral to anterior tibial artery, posterior to extensor tendons.
- **Insert** needle in plane from lateral to medial, using ~3-5 mL anesthetic.

Superficial peroneal nerve block
- **Position** supine, then internally rotate hip to expose lateral lower part of affected leg, or roll patient onto side. The superficial peroneal nerve crosses

through the fascia to become superficial about 12 cm above lateral ankle.
- **Place** the probe anteriorly to the lateral malleolus approximately 10 cm proximal to the ankle. The nerve runs between the peroneus brevis and extensor digitorum longus muscles.
- Using an in plane approach, **inject** 3-5 mL of local anesthesia to surround the nerve.

Sural nerve block
- **Position** supine, with lateral surface of foot exposed.
- **Place** linear probe posterior to lateral malleolus.
- **Identify** branch of saphenous vein and sural nerve, anterior to Achilles tendon.
- **Inject** 3-5 mL local anesthesia around nerve, using an in-plane block.

Distal tibial nerve block
- **Position** supine, with affected leg abducted and externally rotated (ie, frogleg) position, or place position on their side to expose medial malleolus.
- **Place** linear probe posterior to medial malleolus.
- **Identify** posterior tibial nerve, posterior to tibial artery.
- Using either in-plane or out-of-plane technique, **inject** 3-5 mL local anesthetic.

Figure 1. Region of analgesia

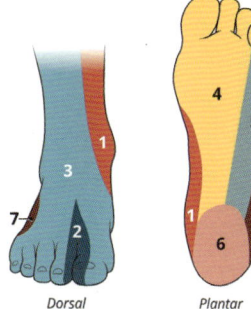

1. Saphenous nerve
2. Deep peroneal nerve
3. Superficial peroneal nerve
4. Medial plantar nerve
5. Lateral plantar nerve
6. Calcaneal branch (tibial nerve)
7. Sural nerve

Dorsal   Plantar

Pearls and Pitfalls

- The ankle is innervated by 5 nerves: saphenous, deep peroneal, superficial peroneal, sural, and distal tibial nerves.
- Although ultrasound can be used with all of these blocks, many clinicians only use it with the deep peroneal nerve block and the distal tibial nerve block due to proximity to vascular structures.
- Blocking the sciatic nerve higher in the leg blocks most of the lower leg, foot, and ankle, except the medial surface of lower leg (saphenous from femoral nerve).

DISTAL TIBIAL NERVE BLOCK

Materials *(adapt to patient, clinician, and site-specific factors/availability)*

Probe	Linear probe
Needle	50 mm, 22 G blunt tip needle; Hyperechoic block needle preferred, tubing optional
Volume of anesthetic	5-10 mL
Other	10 mL syringe; 10 mL sterile saline (for hydrodissection)
	Skin prep and PPE

Region of Analgesia
Anesthetizes the sole / plantar aspect of the foot as well the internal structures of the foot. There is no motor involvement (**Figure 1**).

Indications	Contraindications
• Calcaneal, metatarsal, and phalangeal fracture	• Allergy to local anesthetic
• Sole of foot laceration	• Overlying infection
• Abscess drainage	• Anticoagulation (relative)

Patient Positioning
- Supine, with knee flexed, hip externally rotated, and ankle supported by blankets. Alternately, lateral decubitus position, with affected side down, exposing medial aspect of ankle.

Procedure
1. Sterilize field per local guidelines.
2. **Place** transducer just proximal and posterior to medial malleolus in a transverse orientation. Tibial nerve bundle will be seen just adjacent to tibial artery. Slide probe proximally along nerve, gently tilting to achieve optimal visualization.
3. For **in-plane** approach, enter from **posterior aspect** of leg and gently **advance** toward nerve, placing anesthetic in fascial plane adjacent to nerve.
4. For **out-of-plane** approach, center the probe directly over target nerve, with **needle directed steeply** (60-90° relative to skin), placing anesthetic in fascial plane adjacent to nerve.
5. After negative aspiration, **hydrodissect** nerve away from tissue with sterile saline.
6. Once appropriate hydrodissection is observed, **inject** ~5-10 mL anesthetic.

Pearls and Pitfalls
- The lateral aspect of the foot could be spared and may need additional local anesthetic or an additional block.
- When performing the in-plane technique, slide proximal on the leg so needle does not pass through Achilles tendon.
- The out-of-plane technique may be best because there is not much soft tissue lateral to the nerve in the distal leg. When performing this technique, needle tip visualization can be difficult; ensure lack of intraneural injection.

Figure 1. Region of analgesia

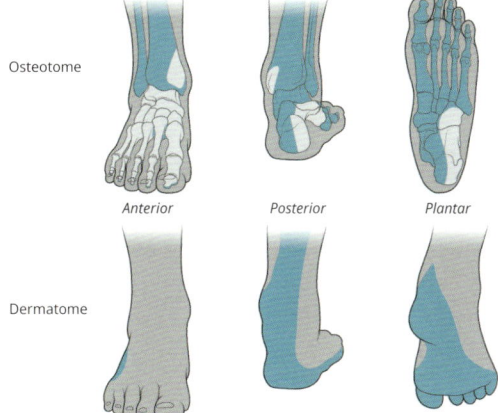

Osteotome — Anterior, Posterior, Plantar

Dermatome

Figure 2 (below, top row): Probe placement
Figure 3 (below, bottom row): Ultrasound anatomy

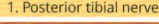

1. Posterior tibial nerve
2. Posterior tibial artery and vein
3. Medial malleolus

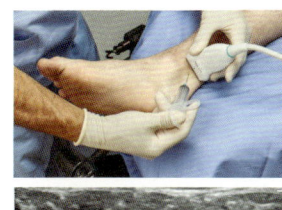
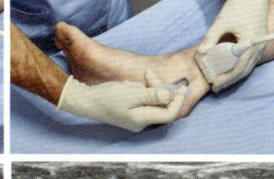
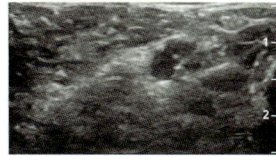
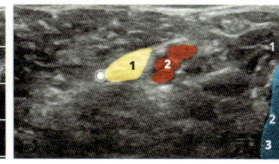

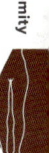

Lower Extremity

Other Musculoskeletal Procedures

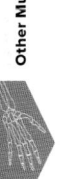

OTHER MUSCULOSKELETAL PROCEDURES

Hematoma Block for Humerus Fractures 76

Hematoma Block for Ankle Fractures 77

Hematoma Block for Wrist Fractures 78

Trigger Point Injection Thoracic & Lumbar Muscles 80

Trigger Point Injection Cervical & Trapezius Muscles 82

Knee Injection 84

Shoulder Injection 86

Hip Injection 88

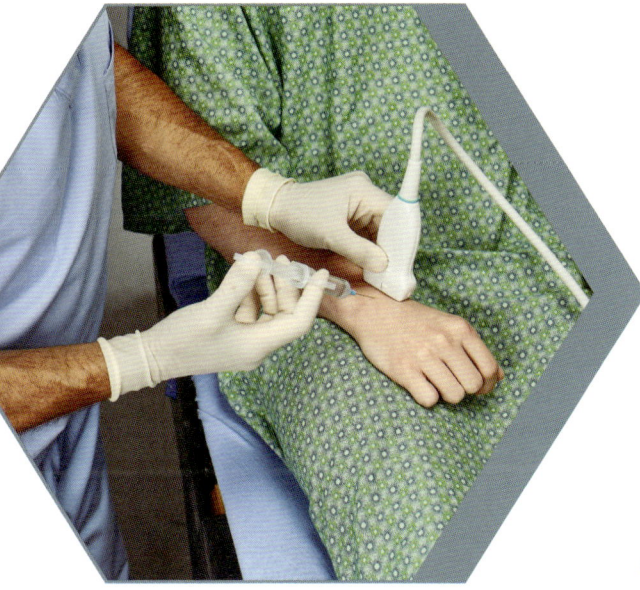

HEMATOMA BLOCK FOR HUMERUS FRACTURES

Materials *(adapt to patient, clinician, and site-specific factors/availability)*

Probe	Optional; high-frequency linear probe, if US is used
Needle	18-22 G, 1.5" long beveled/sharp tip needle
Volume of anesthetic	10-20 mL (bupivacaine relatively contraindicated; lidocaine preferred)
Other	10-20 mL syringe; skin prep and PPE

Region of Analgesia
Anesthetizes the fracture area and some superficial skin around the fracture site. There is no motor involvement.

Indications	Contraindications
• Humerus fractures and/or closed reductions	• Allergy to local anesthetic
	• Overlying infection
	• Anticoagulation (relative)

Patient Positioning
- Seated or supine, with area of fracture accessible for ultrasound and injection

Procedure
1. Sterilize field per local guidelines.
2. **Identify** fracture site by palpation or on ultrasound through direct visualization.
3. **Insert** needle on the lateral aspect of the arm to avoid neurovascular structures. With US, use in-plane approach to guide needle to the fracture site. If using palpation, enter where deformity is palpated and advance until bone is contacted.
4. **Aspirate** blood to confirm needle within hematoma; once confirmed, **inject** anesthetic.

Pearls and Pitfalls
- If not getting blood using blind/palpation technique, consider using US for direct visualization of fracture.
- Do not use bupivacaine; hematoma blocks carry increased risk of LAST.

Figure 1 (below): Ultrasound anatomy

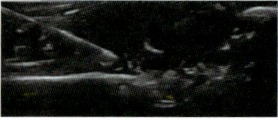
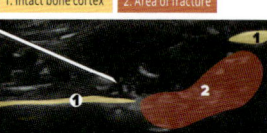

1. Intact bone cortex 2. Area of fracture

HEMATOMA BLOCK FOR ANKLE FRACTURES

Materials *(adapt to patient, clinician, and site-specific factors/availability)*

Probe	Optional; high-frequency linear probe, if US is used
Needle	18-22 G, 1.5" long beveled/sharp tip needle
Volume of anesthetic	10-20 mL (bupivacaine relatively contraindicated; lidocaine preferred)
Other	10-20 mL syringe; skin prep and PPE

Region of Analgesia
Anesthetizes the ankle joint and local structures. There is no motor involvement.

Indications	Contraindications
• Ankle fracture • Closed reduction	• Allergy to local anesthetic • Overlying infection • Anticoagulation (relative)

Patient Positioning
- Seated or supine, medial aspect of ankle exposed to identify tibialis anterior and medial malleolus

Procedure
1. Sterilize field per local guidelines.
2. In **landmark-based technique**, tibial injection is performed between medial malleous and tibialis anterior tendon. If fibular involvement, additional injection can be performed on the anterior-lateral aspect of the lateral malleolus.
3. In **US technique**, start in the transverse orientation between the tibialis anterior and medial malleolus, and scan to visualize the fracture.
4. Under direct visualization, **advance** the needle to the fracture.
5. In both landmark and US-guided approaches, **aspirate** blood to confirm needle within hematoma; once confirmed, **inject** anesthetic.

Figure 1: Needle placement
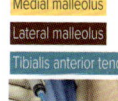
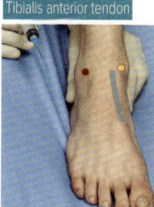

Pearls and Pitfalls
- Reductions can often be performed with hematoma blocks alone, avoiding the need for conscious sedation.
- For displaced fractures, US is rarely required; injection can be done by visualization or palpation.
- If tibia and fibula are both fractured, consider hematoma blocks of both bones.
- Do not use bupivacaine; hematoma blocks carry increased risk of LAST.

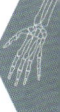

HEMATOMA BLOCK FOR WRIST FRACTURES

Materials *(adapt to patient, clinician, and site-specific factors/availability)*

Probe	Optional; high-frequency linear probe, if US is used
Needle	18-22 G, 1.5" long beveled/sharp tip needle
Volume of anesthetic	10-20 mL (bupivacaine relatively contraindicated; lidocaine preferred)
Other	10-20 mL syringe; skin prep and PPE

Region of Analgesia
Anesthetizes the fracture site and surrounding structures. There is no motor involvement distally.

Indications	Contraindications
• Distal radius and/or ulna fracture/dislocations • Closed reductions	• Allergy to local anesthetic • Overlying infection • Anticoagulation (relative)

Patient Positioning
- Position of comfort, with area of fracture easily accessible, usually with dorsal surface up

Procedure
1. Sterilize field per local guidelines.
2. **Identify** fracture site through palpation and/or ultrasound.
3. **Orient** probe in transverse view to visualize fracture. **Insert** needle on dorsal aspect of wrist, to avoid neurovascular structures. Using an **in-plane** approach, guide needle into fracture site.
4. **Aspirate** blood to confirm needle within hematoma; once confirmed, **inject** anesthetic.

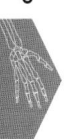

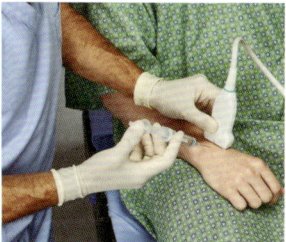

Figure 1 (left): Probe placement *(Note: Photo shows out-of-plane approach; ultrasound is in-plane)*

Figure 2 (below): Ultrasound anatomy

1. Intact bone cortex
2. Area of fracture

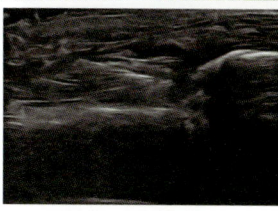
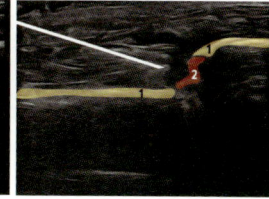

Pearls and Pitfalls

- Reductions can often be performed with hematoma blocks alone, avoiding need for conscious sedation.
- If not getting blood using blind/palpation technique, consider using US for direct visualization of fracture.
- Do not use bupivacaine; hematoma blocks carry increased risk of LAST.

TRIGGER POINT INJECTION (TPI)
THORACIC AND LUMBAR MUSCLES

Materials *(adapt to patient, clinician, and site-specific factors/availability)*

Needle	25-27 G, 1.5" long beveled/sharp tip needle
Volume of anesthetic	10-20 mL
Other	10-20 mL syringe Skin prep and PPE

Region of Analgesia
Anesthetizes the muscle tissue that is directly infiltrated. There is no motor involvement.

Indications	Contraindications
• Back pain	• Allergy to local anesthetic
• Thoracic and lumbar muscle spasm	• Overlying infection

Patient Positioning
- Patient lying prone with back exposed, or seated with back exposed; if seated, have patient lean forward to improve comfort and decrease movement during injections

Procedure
1. Trigger points are focal hyperirritable areas in a band of skeletal muscle. **Identify** trigger points by palpating affected area. Trigger points include areas that have maximal tenderness and are often associated with feeling a tight band or knot of muscle. In general, multiple trigger points are injected during this procedure to obtain maximal pain relief.
2. Sterilize field per local guidelines.
3. **Advance** needle into trigger point, injecting 2-4 mL anesthetic. Increase the efficacy of the trigger point injection (TPI) by fanning injection throughout the area, nearly withdrawing the needle from skin and redirecting it to multiple planes. Repeat for each identified trigger point.
4. On **lumbar** musculature, injections may be done perpendicular to the skin and a 1.5" needle can be advanced to the hub. On **thoracic** musculature, extra attention must be paid to needle depth in order to avoid inadvertent lung puncture. Consider injecting at a **45°-60° angle** and performing shallower injections in areas where there is risk for pneumothorax.
5. **Repeat** injections until all anesthetic is used.

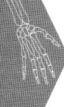

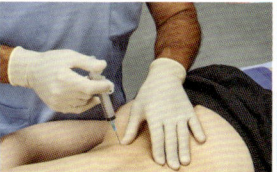
Figure 1: Needle placement, lower back TPI

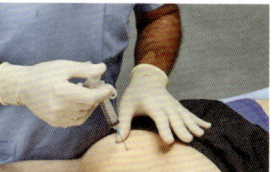
Figure 2: Needle placement, gluteal TPI

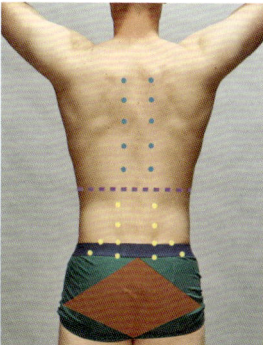
Figure 3 (left): Trigger point areas

- Common thoracic TPI sites
- Line delineates 12th rib, above which there is increased risk of PTX
- Common lumbar TPI sites
- DO NOT INJECT; risk of injury to sciatic nerve

Pearls and Pitfalls

- For additional safety, US can be used to determine depth of pleura and/or peritoneum and avoid accidental pneumothorax or bowel injury.
- Dry needling by rapidly and repeatedly "pistoning" the needle deeper and more shallow (without exiting the skin) around the trigger point may also help. Dry needling can be performed after depositing LA, or without LA. Dry needling can also be done in patients in whom LA is contraindicated or to additional trigger points once you've reached LA limits.

TRIGGER POINT INJECTION (TPI)
CERVICAL AND TRAPEZIUS MUSCLES

Materials *(adapt to patient, clinician, and site-specific factors/availability)*

Needle	25-27 G, 1.5" long beveled/sharp tip needle
Volume of anesthetic	2-3 mL per side if cervical; 2-4 mL per side if trapezius
Other	10-20 mL syringe Skin prep and PPE

Region of Analgesia
Anesthetizes only the muscle tissue that is directly infiltrated. There is no motor involvement.

Indications	Contraindications
• Cervical and trapezius muscle spasm • Headache • Dental pain / facial pain / trigeminal neuralgia	• Allergy to local anesthetic • Overlying infection

Patient Positioning
- **Cervical TPI:** Seated upright, with chin lifted and head facing forward
- **Trapezius TPI:** Seated or prone, with neck and upper back exposed

Procedure
Sterilize field per local guidelines.

Cervical
1. In contrast to other TPIs, these are consistently done in the same area without palpating for trigger points. Palpate cervical spine, identifying area between C4-C6, in mid posterior neck; many clinicians leave thumb in midline for orientation (**Figure 1**).
2. Insert needle into paracervical musculature, 1-2" lateral of midline perpendicular to skin and parallel to the floor (inferior angling risks pneumothorax).
3. Needle is inserted 1-1.5" in a smooth motion (contrary to other trigger points, do not join injection or perform dry needling).
4. Aspirate, then inject 2-3 mL anesthetic.
5. Cervical TPIs are typically done as a single shot, bilaterally.
6. Cervical TPIs are often combined with occipital nerve blocks for headache relief.

Trapezius
1. Trigger points are focal hyperirritable areas in a band of skeletal muscle. Identify trigger points by palpating the affected area. Trigger points include areas of maximal tenderness and are often associated with feeling a tight band or knot of muscle.
2. Insert needle at 45°-60° angle relative to the skin, being cautious of depth to reduce risk of inadvertent pneumothorax.
3. Can pinch trapezius trigger points between 4 fingers and thumb and direct the needle between the fingers and thumb into the trigger point (**Figure 2**). This affords better needle control and decreased PTX risk, but increases risk of needle stick injury.
4. Inject 2-4 mL anesthetic, fanning injection throughout the area.
5. Repeat for each identified trigger point.

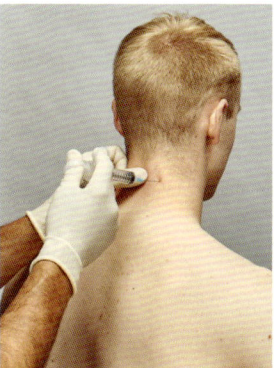
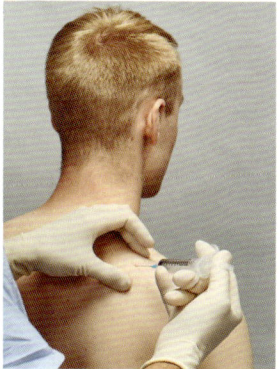

Figure 1: Needle placement, paracervical TPI

Figure 2: Needle placement, trapezius TPI

Figure 3 (left): Trigger point areas

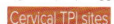
Cervical TPI sites

Common trapezius TPI sites

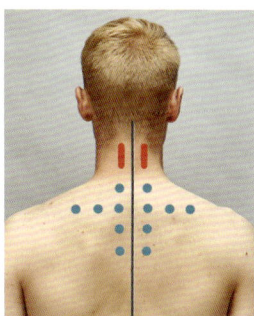

Pearls and Pitfalls

- Cervical and trapezius TPIs both carry risk of pneumothorax; be cognizant of needle angles and consent patients to this risk.
- Cervical TPI has shown benefit for facial and dental pain, in addition to headache and neck pain.
- For additional safety, US can be used to determine depth of pleura and avoid accidental pneumothorax when performing trapezius or cervical TPIs.

Other Musculoskeletal Procedures

KNEE INJECTION

Materials *(adapt to patient, clinician, and site-specific factors/availability)*

Probe	Optional; high-frequency linear probe, if US is used
Needle	18-22 G, 1.5" long beveled/sharp tip needle
Volume of anesthetic	10 mL; consider addition of 40 mg/1 mL of triamcinolone to LA
Other	10 mL syringe Full sterile prep and PPE

Region of Analgesia
Local anesthesia at injection site is used to anesthetize the skin, subdermal tissue, and the joint capsule, although additional anesthetic may be injected into the articular space for general knee joint analgesia if desired. There is no motor involvement.

Indications	Contraindications
• Diagnosis of joint infection or inflammatory process, such as gout • Therapeutic intra-articular injections	• Allergy to local anesthetic • Overlying infection • Known bacteremia (relative) • Anticoagulation (relative)

Patient Positioning
- Supine or seated, with affected knee slightly flexed and positioned closest to operator; US should be on opposite side of patient, screen facing operator.

Procedure
1. **Sterilize** field per local guidelines. Full sterile prep with sterile gloves, probe cover, and drape is recommended.
2. **Place** linear transducer in prepatellar fossa in longitudinal direction, with probe marker positioned caudally.
3. **Identify** patella, then slide probe cephalad to visualize patella, femur, quadriceps femoris tendon, and fat pad.
4. An effusion will appear as an anechoic fluid collection deep to fat pad.
5. For anesthetic injection, a lateral to medial in-plane technique is recommended.
6. With linear probe in prepatellar fossa, **rotate** probe marker (clockwise) to patient's right to obtain a transverse view of the prepatellar space.
7. **Inject** a small amount of local anesthetic to create skin wheal just lateral to US transducer (the projected entry point for joint arthrocentesis), making sure to anesthetize down to the joint capsule.
8. Using 10 mL (or larger) syringe attached to 18 G needle, **enter** the skin in plane at site of anesthesia, just lateral to the probe at a shallow angle.
9. The needle should traverse between the iliotibial band (superiorly) and vastus lateralis (inferiorly) without risk for vascular puncture; **advance** directly under the probe for visualization of the needle.

10. Gently **aspirate** synovial fluid, with needle tip being visualized within the fluid collection, to confirm entrance into the joint space.
11. **Inject** anesthetic.

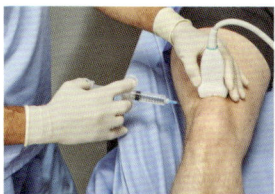

Figure 1 (left): Probe placement (full sterile prep excluded to show needle placement)
Figure 2 (below): Ultrasound anatomy
A. Longitudinal view; B. Transverse view

1. Patella
2. Quadriceps tendon
3. Femur

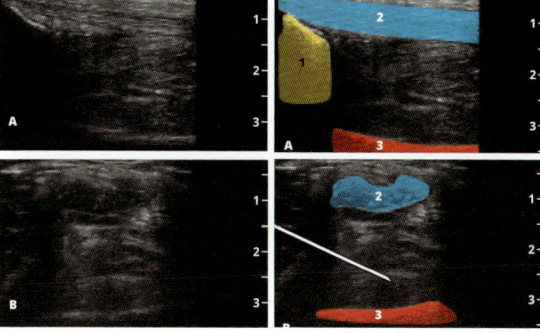

Pearls and Pitfalls

- Evaluate with US prior to sterilizing your field.
- Iodine can be transferred into joint space and produce an inflammatory reaction. If used, wipe off in a sterile fashion prior to procedure, or use alternative skin prep.
- Ultrasound the non-affected suprapatellar space for comparison.
- Consider alternate approach with significant pain or inability to aspirate synovial fluid ("dry tap").
- The synovial membrane, articular capsule, and periosteum have extensive nerve fiber supply and are exceptionally sensitive.

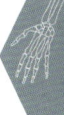

SHOULDER INJECTION

Materials *(adapt to patient, clinician, and site-specific factors/availability)*

Probe	Optional; high-frequency linear probe, if US is used
Needle	18-22 G, long beveled/sharp tip needle or 22 G, 3.5" spinal needle
Volume of anesthetic	10-20 mL; consider addition of 40 mg/1 mL of triamcinolone to LA
Other	10-20 mL syringe Full sterile prep and PPE *Optional: 1-2 mL 1% lidocaine in separate syringe for skin wheal*

Region of Analgesia
Intra-articular glenohumeral joint injection provides anesthesia to the entire shoulder joint. There is no motor involvement.

Indications	Contraindications
• Diagnosis of joint infection or inflammatory process, such as gout • Therapeutic intra-articular injections • Anesthesia for closed shoulder reduction	• Allergy to local anesthetic • Overlying infection • Known bacteremia (relative) • Anticoagulation (relative)

Patient Positioning
- Seated, facing away from operator

Procedure
1. **Sterilize** field per local guidelines. Full sterile prep with sterile gloves, probe cover and drape is recommended.
2. Place US system in front of the patient. **Palpate** the patient's scapular spine and to **identify** the basic surface anatomy.
3. Using the low-frequency curvilinear or linear probe with probe marker toward patient's left, align the probe parallel to bed. **Place** probe just inferior to scapular spine and slowly move laterally until humeral head, glenohumeral joint, and scapular spine are clearly visualized (**Figure 1**).
4. Using M-mode marker or needle guidance line, center the glenohumeral joint on screen (**Figure 2**).
5. **Insert** needle tip parallel to probe, just under scapular spine. While advancing needle, gently **aspirate** until synovial fluid is obtained. If performing intra-articular analgesia, **inject** preferred anesthetic at this point. Using 10 mL (or larger) syringe attached to 18 G needle, enter skin in plane at site of anesthesia, just lateral to probe, at a shallow angle.

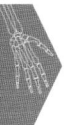

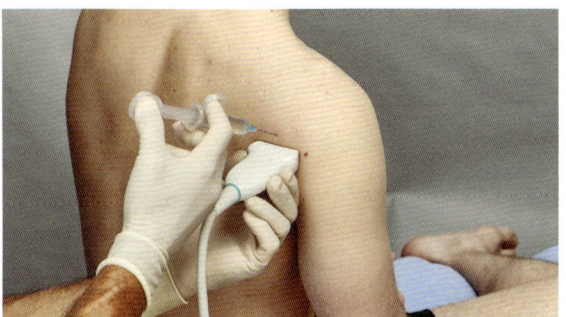

Figure 1 (above): Probe placement for **out-of-plane injection** (full sterile prep excluded to show needle placement)
Figure 2 (below): Ultrasound anatomy showing in-plane lateral needle approach

1. Deltoid
2. Glenoid
3. Infraspinatus muscle
4. Humeral head

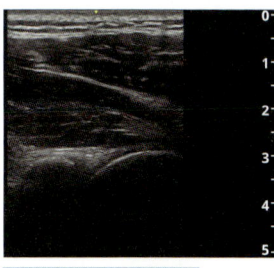
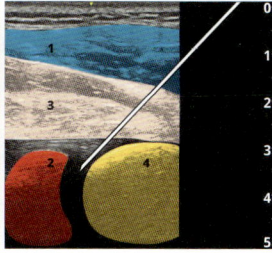

Pearls and Pitfalls

- Evaluate with US prior to sterilizing your field.
- Iodine can be transferred into joint space and produce an inflammatory reaction. If used, wipe off in a sterile fashion prior to procedure, or use alternative skin prep.
- Compare affected shoulder to unaffected shoulder to identify smaller effusions.
- An in-plane approach can also be used by advancing the needle from lateral to medial until you enter the glenohumeral joint.
- US can help identify dislocations and/or confirm successful joint reductions.

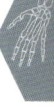

HIP INJECTION

Materials *(adapt to patient, clinician, and site-specific factors/availability)*

Probe	Curvilinear or high-frequency linear probe for shallower depth
Needle	22 G, 3.5-5" spinal needle
Volume of anesthetic	3-10 mL; consider addition of 40 mg/1 mL of triamcinolone to LA
Other	10 mL syringe Full sterile prep and PPE

Region of Analgesia

Local anesthesia at injection site anesthetizes skin and subdermal tissue; injection provides analgesia to the hip joint. There is no motor involvement.

Indications	Contraindications
• Diagnosis of joint infection or inflammatory process, such as gout • Therapeutic intra-articular injections	• Allergy to local anesthetic • Overlying infection • Known bacteremia (relative) • Anticoagulation (relative)

Patient Positioning

- Supine, with knee slightly flexed and hip mildly internally rotated. US machine should be on opposite side, with screen facing operator.

Procedure

1. **Sterilize** field per local guidelines. Full sterile prep with sterile gloves, probe cover, and drape is recommended.
2. **Palpate** femoral artery and place transducer in a parallel plane to inguinal ligament so vessels are visualized, with probe marker toward patient's right side.
3. **Rotate** probe so probe marker points to umbilicus.
4. **Visualize** the femoral head and neck, acetabulum, iliofemoral ligament and anterior synovial recess (**Figure 2**).
5. Sterilize field per local guidelines, sterile drape open at anterior affected hip, probe fitted with sterile sheath.
6. Image affected hip as above, and **inject** 3-5 mL local anesthetic about 1 cm caudal to probe.
7. Using an in-plane technique, enter skin at 30° angle, aiming at anterior recess (**Figure 1**).
8. **Advance** needle slowly until tip passes under ligament, then gently **aspirate** synovial fluid.

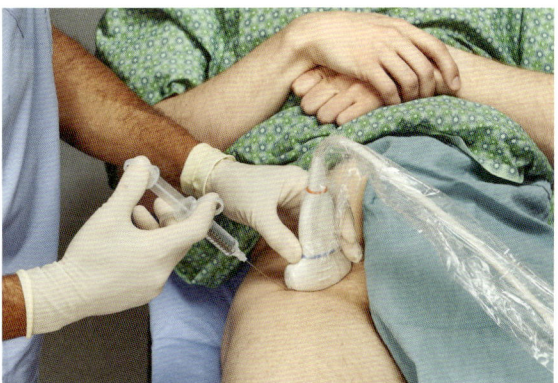

Figure 1 (above): Probe placement (full sterile prep excluded to show needle placement)
Figure 2 (below): Ultrasound anatomy

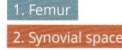

1. Femur
2. Synovial space

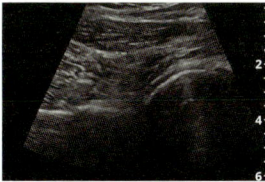
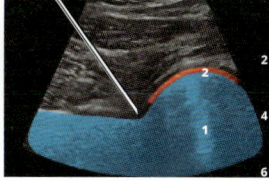

Pearls and Pitfalls

- Evaluate with US prior to sterilizing your field.
- Iodine can be transferred into joint space and produce an inflammatory reaction. If used, wipe off in a sterile fashion prior to procedure, or use alternative skin prep.
- Evaluate the opposite side to compare the amount of fluid.
- Femoral vessels are medial and should be identified prior to arthrocentesis.
- Classic criterion for hip effusion in an adult is an anechoic or hypoechoic fluid stripe > 5 mm located under the iliofemoral ligament, or 2 mm of asymmetry as compared to the unaffected hip.

Other Musculoskeletal Procedures

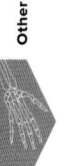

ADMINISTRATION/OPERATIONS

What Is Advanced Analgesia? 92

Evidence of Benefit 92

How to Implement Regional Anesthesia Training 93

Reimbursement 97

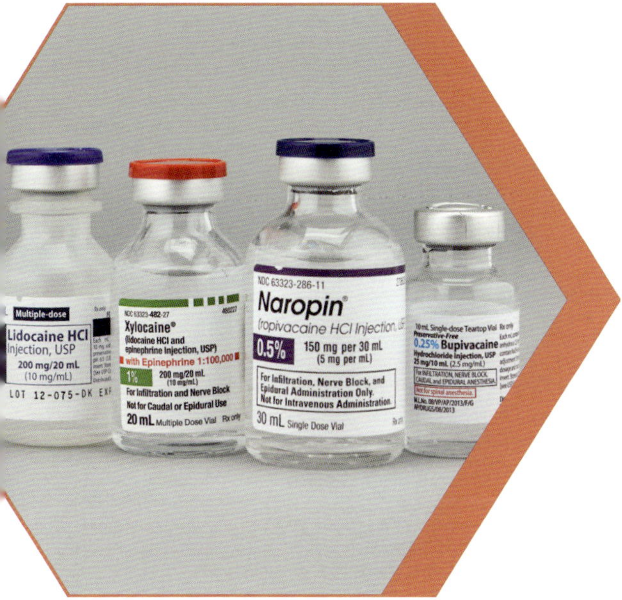

WHAT IS ADVANCED ANALGESIA?

Advanced analgesia integrates the best evidence-based practices into an easily understandable and applicable framework that emphasizes optimal patient care. Regional analgesia is an important tool in the advanced management of pain in the emergency department. RA as a practice holds significant benefits in terms of length of stay, patient satisfaction, and morbidity and mortality. Through mastery of the pillars of pain management, clinicians will find themselves less dependent on opioid analgesics and more capable of providing patients with a multimodal pain plan. The importance of decreasing opioid utilization, especially in the context of our current opioid crisis, cannot be overstated.

Depending on the nerve or field block, anesthesia can be achieved over large areas. Blocks can be performed to help augment pain control or provide complete analgesia to facilitate ED-based procedures including laceration repair, incision and drainage, central line placement, chest tube placement, and fracture/dislocation reduction among others.

Although some nerve blocks may be performed by landmark techniques (ie, dental blocks, wrist blocks), ultrasound guidance has increased success and safety of RA.

In addition, regional and procedural analgesia represent an area of medicine where optimal care is recognized by payors, including state and federal programs. Adding RA to the practice of emergency medicine makes sense for patients and is financially viable for clinicians and their groups.

EVIDENCE OF BENEFIT

Regional anesthesia has emerged as an effective alternative to opioid medications for treating pain in the ED. Its safety and overall efficacy in the ED has been proven through multiple investigations. As such, it is rapidly becoming a core tool in the emergency physician's management of pain at the bedside. The role of RA in the management of pain is also increasingly being integrated into guidelines and clinical workflows nationwide. RA has been endorsed by the American College of Surgeons as best practice in the management of trauma patients and required for credentialed trauma centers.

In the ED setting, RA has been shown to have multiple patient-centered benefits:
- Decreased length of stay
- Reduction in need for procedural sedation
- Reduction in ED/hospital opioid requirements
- Increased overall patient satisfaction compared to other methods of pain control
- May decrease mortality for hip and rib fractures

In addition, RA is reimbursed and (most important) provides emergency clinicians with the gratification of seeing patients improve right before their eyes.

In general, performing RA with ultrasound guidance improves the success rate over landmark-based approaches and decreases the time to onset of sensory blockade, anesthetic volume requirement, block performance time, and rate of complications.

Ultrasound-guided regional anesthesia (UGRA) is increasingly being performed in academic emergency medicine centers throughout the country, with 84% of institutions reporting performance of these procedures in early 2023.

HOW TO IMPLEMENT REGIONAL ANESTHESIA TRAINING

Coordinate with hospital leadership and other departments

Initiate meetings with all pertinent stakeholders and hospital leadership to develop a clear interdepartmental plan for optimal pain control utilizing RA. Buy-in is required from multiple departments: anesthesia, orthopedics, surgery, and other services that may see patients who receive blocks in the ED. Coordination is essential to optimize care and reduce confusion and potential patient harms.

Common concerns from specialists include documentation, masking of the neurologic exam, compartment syndrome, and peripheral nerve injury. Address these valid concerns through creating good policies, procedures, and training.

Establish protocols with pharmacy to provide access to local anesthetics, adjuvants and intralipid. It is recommended that intralipid be available outside of automated medication dispensing systems. Many departments have a "block box" containing all essential medications that can be taken to the bedside and then inventoried by protocol; this can drastically speed up workflow.

Block Box

A user-based design approach will reduce barriers needed to perform RA blocks. Keep all supplies needed for performing RA blocks in one location (ie, tray, bag, or cart) to streamline the process.

A block cart should be mobile, well-organized, and routinely restocked. It should contain all equipment needed to perform RA blocks (skin preps, protective adhesive barriers, needles/block needles, syringes, sterile gel, marking pens), in addition to a diverse array of local anesthetics, adjuncts, and intralipid in case of rare but life-threatening complications.

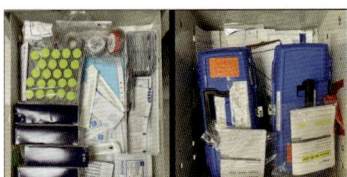
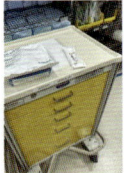

Figure 1 (left): Block box drawer   Figure 2 (right): Block box cart

Documentation Templates

Documentation of an RA block is required for communication to other providers/services as well as for accurate and consistent billing.

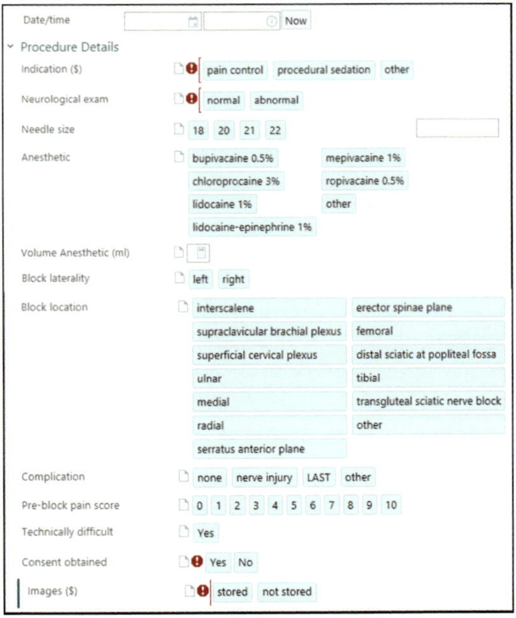

Date/time		
Procedure Details		
Indication ($)	pain control	procedural sedation	other
Neurological exam	normal	abnormal
Needle size	18	20	21	22
Anesthetic	bupivacaine 0.5%	mepivacaine 1%
	chloroprocaine 3%	ropivacaine 0.5%
	lidocaine 1%	other
	lidocaine-epinephrine 1%	
Volume Anesthetic (ml)		
Block laterality	left	right
Block location	interscalene	erector spinae plane
	supraclavicular brachial plexus	femoral
	superficial cervical plexus	distal sciatic at popliteal fossa
	ulnar	tibial
	medial	transgluteal sciatic nerve block
	radial	other
	serratus anterior plane	
Complication	none	nerve injury	LAST	other
Pre-block pain score	0 1 2 3 4 5 6 7 8 9 10
Technically difficult	Yes
Consent obtained	Yes	No
Images ($)	stored	not stored

Templated notes in the electronic medical record allow the clinician to document important information, including:
- Indication for the block
- Block type
- Laterality
- Anesthetic type and amount used
- Complications
- Time the block was performed

Identify a Clinical Champion, Develop Skills

Identify a clinical champion to develop expertise and serve as a resource to others learning new skills. The clinical champion can obtain required skills several ways:
- **Use local resources:** RA is often performed by anesthesiologists perioperatively. Develop partnerships with anesthesiology and surgery to learn skills under the guidance of an experienced, local practitioner. This also allows the clinical champion to determine the equipment, medications, and tools already used in their hospital for RA in order to build the "block box."
- **Attend a national course on regional analgesia:** There are courses run by anesthesiology as well as EM. The hands-on component (either in simulation or cadavers) should be a central aspect of the course.
- **Use written and online resources:** There are multiple textbooks on regional analgesia. The champion's learning can also be supplemented and refreshed via numerous online resources.

Educate Physician/Practice Group

Once the RA clinical champion has acquired the skills to perform blocks, s/he will need to establish a training pathway for other physicians at the institution. Scaling to all clinicians is often the most challenging step. Clinicians or hospitals can consider sending their physicians to national courses or hosting local courses using specialists or consultants.

Local champions can identify 1-2 high-yield RA blocks. The easiest to teach and most pertinent RA blocks include: fascia iliaca/femoral nerve block for hip fractures, serratus anterior or erector spinae blocks for rib fractures and thoracic injuries, and forearm nerve blocks for hand injuries. Limit the number of RA blocks in the initial training of novice staff to allow learners to focus on the general principles of RA as well as good needling techniques.

Tailor training to the learners' experience with procedural ultrasound. Learners with minimal experience may benefit from the use of needle trainer devices, which can either be purchased or created at home using household supplies. Programs can also use existing hospital simulation centers if available.

The RA clinical champion should do clinical hands-on training on shift. Learners can consider scheduling training shifts in the ED with the RA clinical champion to perform blocks.

Also consider establishing agreements with anesthesia to allow learning from anesthesiologists performing RA blocks in the perioperative setting.

Get Credentialed

In 2021, the American College of Emergency Physicians (ACEP) issued a policy statement specific to RA programs, affirming that ED-provider-performed RA blocks are not only within the scope of EM, but also are a "core component" of pain control for ED patients, pointing to their rising role as the new standard of care for acutely ill or injured patients. Landmark-based nerve blocks have long been a part of the ACGME's EM residency education requirement (Milestones 1.0), with ultrasound guidance improving their safety profile. According to an ACEP policy statement reaffirmed in 2020, the provider with emergency ultrasound privileges needs no outside certification to perform RA blocks. While this may seem surprising to some, note that no other clinical procedure requires special external certification: for example, central venous access or intubation, which follow a similar historical path of being brought into EM after initially exclusively being performed by anesthesia or critical care specialists. As with EM, anesthesia physicians also require no additional certification to perform nerve blocks. All physicians are encouraged to know if RA is already covered in their hospital credentialing; if it is not, then this should be added prior to broad adoption of RA by emergency clinicians.

Initiating and updating emergency physicians' RA block privileges can be done safely via the standard intradepartmental credentialing approval process. As of 2023, ACEP guidelines require individuals obtaining initial credentialing to complete the training and proof of competency determined by their own ED. The guidelines suggest an approximate threshold of 10 with new ultrasound procedures that build upon existing procedural skills; for example, 10 transvaginal ultrasounds for those who already perform POCUS, rather than the usual threshold of 25 when learning a new application of ultrasound. For reference, The American Institute of Ultrasound in Medicine recommends anesthesiologists perform 20 RA blocks per year to maintain competence.

REIMBURSEMENT

Regional analgesia presents an opportunity to provide better care for patients, and also reimbursable care for physician and physician groups. While there is direct reimbursement for procedures performed by emergency physicians, the far greater benefit to the health system and patients is decreased costs from decreased length of stay, decreased morbidity and mortality, and improved patient satisfaction.

RVU Table (based on 2023 Medicare payment rates)
Please see the next page for a reimbursement reference table.
- Medicare payment = RVU x current Medicare conversion factor ($33.887 for 2023).
- Medicaid rates typically pay between 50-80% of Medicare.
- Private insurance typically pays 1.25-10 times Medicare rates.
- Most insurers and Medicare decrease the second and subsequent procedures performed on the same day by 50-75% reimbursement of the fee schedule. Modifier 51 is appended to the CPT code.
- The work RVU is only one portion of the total RVU generated. The total RVU will depend on the practice expense RVU, malpractice expense RVU and work RVU, all of which undergo a geographic practice cost index (GPCI) adjustment.
- To calculate the Total RVU for your region, multiply Total RVU X (GPCI for your region).

Notes: Table 7.1. RA Reimbursement, 2023

+ (Superficial) Cervical Plexus block CPT code 64413 was deleted Jan. 1, 2023, and does not have an applicable CPT. Coders are instructed to use 64999 which is "Other nervous system procedure" and bills 0 RVU. Many nerve block procedures are not listed under a formal CPT code. The code 64450, "other peripheral nerve or branch" should be used in most of these scenarios.

* For the complete forearm and hand blocks, the RVUs will be decreased as there are multiple procedures. Modifier 51 will be appended to the second two blocks, resulting in 50% decrease in reimbursement of those two.

** The use of ultrasound for guidance is bundled for the following blocks (of the ones listed above) and is not separately reported: brachial plexus, axillary, femoral (PENG, FI, adductor canal), TAP. When US is a separate procedure, Modifier 51 is appended, resulting in 50% decrease in reimbursement.

Notes

These CPT codes are referring to "single shot" as opposed to continuous infusion through a temporary catheter. There are different codes for continuous infusion blocks.

For hematoma blocks, use the joint injection code if in the joint, and use the forearm or ankle block if in the shaft.

CPT information obtained from AMA 2023 CPT Codebook.

RVU information obtained from CMS Physician Fee Schedule released Jan. 5, 2023.

Table 7.1. RA Reimbursement, 2023

BLOCK	Work RVU /Medicare	Total RVU/ Medicare
Head and Neck		
Trigeminal Nerve Block (64400)	0.75/$25.42	1.50/$50.83
Superficial Cervical Plexus Block (64999)	+	+
Greater Auricular Nerve Block (64450)	0.75/$25.42	1.24/$42.02
Occipital Nerve Block (64405)	0.94/$31.85	1.57/$53.20
Upper Extremity		
Interscalene brachial plexus block (64415)	1.50/$50.83	2.05/$69.47
Supraclavicular brachial plexus block (64415)	1.50/$50.83	2.05/$69.47
Suprascapular Block (64418)	1.1/$37.28	1.65/$55.91
Ulnar Nerve Block (64450)	0.75/$25.42	1.24/$42.02
Radial Nerve Block (64450)	0.75/$25.42	1.24/$42.02
Median Nerve Block (64450)	0.75/$25.42	1.24/$42.02
Complete Forearm Nerve block (All 3 nerves)	1.5/$50.84*	2.48/$84.04*
Landmark based Hand Block (All 3 nerves)	1.5/$50.84*	2.48/$84.04*
Torso / Abdomen		
Serratus Anterior Block (64450)	0.75/$25.42	1.24/$42.02
PECS I Block (64450)	0.75/$25.42	1.24/$42.02
PECS II Block	0.75/$25.42	1.24/$42.02
Erector Spinae Block	0.75/$25.42	1.24/$42.02
TAP Block unilateral (64486)	1.27/$43.04	1.63/$55.24
TAP Blocks bilateral (64488)	1.6/$54.21	2.02/$68.45
PENG Block (64447)	1.34/$45.41	1.86/$63.03
Axillary Nerve Block (64417)	1.31/$44.37	1.87/$63.37

Lower Extremity		
Fascia Iliaca Block (64447)	1.34/$45.41	1.86/$63.03
Femoral Nerve Block (64447)	1.34/$45.41	1.86/$63.03
Adductor Canal Block	1.34/$45.41	1.86/$63.03
Popliteal Block (64445)	1.39/$47.10	2.17/$73.53
Ankle Block/Injection (20605)	0.68/$23.04	1.10/$37.28
Ankle Block/Injection with US (20606)	1.0/$33.89	1.54/$52.19
Posterior Tibial nerve block	0.75/$25.42	1.24/$42.02
Joint or Bursa Injections		
*Same code and reimbursement for the physician regardless of injection or aspiration		
Knees, Hip, Shoulder (20610)	0.79/$26.77	1.34/$45.41
Knees, Hip, Shoulder with US (20611)	1.10/$37.28	1.78/$60.32
Ankle, wrist, elbow, AC, TMJ (20605)	0.68/$23.04	1.54/$52.19
Ankle, wrist, elbow, AC, TMJ with US (20606)	1.0/$33.89	1.54/$52.19
Trigger Point Injections		
Injection 1 or 2 named muscles (20552)	0.66/$22.37	1.10/$37.28
Injection 3 or more named muscles (20553)	0.75/$25.41	1.26/$42.70
Dry Needling/Acupuncture 1 or 2 named muscles (20560)	0.32/$10.84	0.44/$14.91
Dry Needling/Acupuncture 3 or more named muscles	0.48/$16.26	0.62/$21.00
ULTRASOUND for nerve blocks		
**US for nerve block (76942–51)	0.34/$11.52	0.42/$14.23

APPENDIX

REFERENCES

Local Anesthetic Choice
- Brummett CM, Williams BA. Additives to local anesthetics for peripheral nerve blockade. *Int Anesthesiol Clin.* 2011;49(4):104-116.
- Gropper MA, Miller RD. Miller's Anesthesia. 9th ed. Philadelphia, PA: Elsevier; 2020.
- Huynh TM, Marret E, Bonnet F. Combination of dexamethasone and local anaesthetic solution in peripheral nerve blocks: A meta-analysis of randomised controlled trials. *Eur J Anaesthesiol.* 2015;32(11):751-758.
- Kirkham KR, Jacot-Guillarmod A, Albrecht E. Optimal Dose of Perineural Dexamethasone to Prolong Analgesia After Brachial Plexus Blockade: A Systematic Review and Meta-analysis. *Anesth Analg.* 2018;126(1):270-279.
- Knezevic NN, Anantamongkol U, Candido KD. Perineural dexamethasone added to local anesthesia for brachial plexus block improves pain but delays block onset and motor blockade recovery. *Pain Physician.* 2015;18(1):1-14.
- Pehora C, Pearson AM, Kaushal A, Crawford MW, Johnston B. Dexamethasone as an adjuvant to peripheral nerve block. *Cochrane Database Syst Rev.* 2017;11(11):CD011770.
- Popitz-Bergez FA, Leeson S, Thalhammer JG, Strichartz GR. Intraneural lidocaine uptake compared with analgesic differences between pregnant and nonpregnant rats. *Reg Anesth.* 1997;22(4):363-371.
- Taylor A, McLeod G. Basic pharmacology of local anaesthetics [published correction appears in BJA Educ. 2020 Apr;20(4):140]. *BJA Educ.* 2020;20(2):34-41.

Risks of Regional Anesthesia (RA)
- Auroy Y, Benhamou D, Bargues L, et al. Major complications of regional anesthesia in France: The SOS Regional Anesthesia Hotline Service [published correction appears in Anesthesiology. 2003 Feb;98(2):595. Mercier Frédéric [corrected to Mercier Frédéric J]]. *Anesthesiology.* 2002;97(5):1274-1280.
- Hebl JR. The importance and implications of aseptic techniques during regional anesthesia. *Reg Anesth Pain Med.* 2006;31(4):311-323.
- Neal JM, Barrington MJ, Brull R, et al. The Second ASRA Practice Advisory on Neurologic Complications Associated With Regional Anesthesia and Pain Medicine: Executive Summary 2015. *Reg Anesth Pain Med.* 2015;40(5):401-430.
- Tucker RV, Peterson WJ, Mink JT, et al. Defining an Ultrasound-guided Regional Anesthesia Curriculum for Emergency Medicine. *AEM Educ Train.* 2020;5(3):e10557.

Local Anesthetic Systemic Toxicity (LAST)
- Arumugam S, Contino V, Kolli S. Local Anesthetic Systemic Toxicity (LAST) – a Review and Update. *Curr Anesthesiol Rep.* 2020;10:218–226.
- Ciechanowicz S, Patil V. Lipid emulsion for local anesthetic systemic toxicity. *Anesthesiol Res Pract.* 2012;2012:131784.
- Long B, Chavez S, Gottlieb M, Montrief T, Brady WJ. Local anesthetic systemic toxicity: A narrative review for emergency clinicians. *Am J Emerg Med.* 2022;59:42-48.

Superficial Cervical Plexus Block
- Gürkan Y, Taş Z, Toker K, Solak M. Ultrasound guided bilateral cervical plexus block reduces postoperative opioid consumption following thyroid surgery. *J Clin Monit Comput.* 2015;29(5):579-584.
- Kende P, Wadewale M, Mathai P, Landge J, Desai H, Nimma V. Role of Superficial Cervical Plexus Nerve Block as an Adjuvant to Local Anesthesia in the Maxillofacial Surgical Practice. *J Oral Maxillofac Surg.* 2021;79(11):2247-2256.
- Li J, Szabova A. Ultrasound-Guided Nerve Blocks in the Head and Neck for Chronic Pain Management: The Anatomy, Sonoanatomy, and Procedure. *Pain Physician.* 2021;24(8):533–548.
- Pandit JJ, Bree S, Dillon P, Elcock D, McLaren ID, Crider B. A Comparison of Superficial Versus Combined (Superficial and Deep) Cervical Plexus Block for Carotid Endarterectomy: A Prospective, Randomized Study. *Anesthesia & Analgesia.* 2000;91(4):781-786.
- Tran DQH, Dugani S, Finlayson RJ. A Randomized Comparison Between Ultrasound-Guided and Landmark-Based Superficial Cervical Plexus Block. *Reg Anesth Pain Med.* 2010;35(6):539-543.
- Winnie AP, Ramamurthy S, Durrani Z, Radonjic R. Interscalene Cervical Plexus Block: A Single-Injection Technic. *Anesthesia & Analgesia.* 1975;54(3):370-375.

Greater Auricular Nerve Block
- Chang K, Wu W, Özçakar L. Greater Auricular Nerve Entrapment/Block in a Patient With Postinfectious Stiff Neck: Imaging and Guidance With Ultrasound. *Pain Pract*. 2020;20(3):336-337.
- Ellison MB, Howell S, Heiraty P, Wilson C, Shepherd J, Ellison PR. A Novel Approach to Postoperative Ear Pain — Greater Auricular Nerve Block Catheter: A Case Report. *A&A Practice*. 2020;14(1):21-24.
- Flores S, Herring AA. Ultrasound-guided Greater Auricular Nerve Block for Emergency Department Ear Laceration and Ear Abscess Drainage. *J Emerg Med*. 2016;50(4):651-655.
- Ritchie MK, Wilson CA, Grose BW, Ranganathan P, Howell SM, Ellison MB. Ultrasound-Guided Greater Auricular Nerve Block as Sole Anesthetic for Ear Surgery. *Clinics and Practice*. 2016;6(2):856.

Occipital Nerve Block
- Ward JB. Greater Occipital Nerve Block. *Semin Neurol*. 2003;23(1):059-062.
- Natsis K, Baraliakos X, Appell HJ, Tsikaras P, Gigis I, Koebke J. The course of the greater occipital nerve in the suboccipital region: A proposal for setting landmarks for local anesthesia in patients with occipital neuralgia. *Clin Anat*. 2006;19(4):332-336.
- Ryu JH, Shim JH, Yeom JH, Shin WJ, Cho SY, Jeon WJ. Ultrasound-guided greater occipital nerve block with botulinum toxin for patients with chronic headache in the occipital area: a randomized controlled trial. *Korean J Anesthesiol*. 2019;72(5):479-485.
- Vanterpool SG, Heidel RE, Rejoub LR. Targeting Occipital Headache Pain: Preliminary Data Supporting an Alternative Approach to Occipital Nerve Block. *Clin J Pain*. 2020;36(4):289-295.
- Velásquez-Rimachi V, Chachaima-Mar J, Cárdenas-Baltazar EC, et al. Greater occipital nerve block for chronic migraine patients: A meta-analysis. *Acta Neuro Scandinavica*. Published online June 21, 2022:ane.13634.

Supraorbital Nerve Block
- Betz D, Fane K. Mental Nerve Block. In: StatPearls. StatPearls Publishing; 2022. http://www.ncbi.nlm.nih.gov/books/NBK482243/. Accessed July 9, 2022.
- Nanayakkara D, Manawaratne R, Sampath H, Vadysinghe A, Peiris R. Supraorbital nerve exits: positional variations and localization relative to surgical landmarks. *Anat Cell Biol*. 2018;51(1):19.
- Napier A, De Jesus O, Taylor A. Supraorbital Nerve Block. In: StatPearls. StatPearls Publishing; 2022. http://www.ncbi.nlm.nih.gov/books/NBK536937/. Accessed July 11, 2022.
- Nardi NM, Alvarado AC, Schaefer TJ. Infraorbital Nerve Block. In: StatPearls. StatPearls Publishing; 2022. http://www.ncbi.nlm.nih.gov/books/NBK499881/. Accessed July 9, 2022.
- Wongkietkachorn A, Surakunprapha P, Wongkietkachorn N, Wongkietkachorn S. Safe Zone for Infraorbital Nerve Block. *Plastic and Reconstructive Surgery*. 2019;144(4):709e-710e.

PECS I and II Block
- Blanco R. The 'pecs block': a novel technique for providing analgesia after breast surgery: Correspondence. *Anaesthesia*. 2011;66(9):847-848.
- Chin KJ, Versyck B, Pawa A. Ultrasound-guided fascial plane blocks of the chest wall: a state-of-the-art review. *Anaesthesia*. 2021;76(S1):110-126.
- Jack JM, McLellan E, Versyck B, Englesakis MF, Chin KJ. The role of serratus anterior plane and pectoral nerves blocks in cardiac surgery, thoracic surgery and trauma: a qualitative systematic review. *Anaesthesia*. 2020;75(10):1372-1385.
- Pawa A, Wight J, Onwochei DN, et al. Combined thoracic paravertebral and pectoral nerve blocks for breast surgery under sedation: a prospective observational case series. *Anaesthesia*. 2018;73(4):438-443.

Serratus Anterior Plane Block
- Ahuja D, Biswas S, Bharati S. Regarding the paper published "Serratus anterior plane block: Anatomical landmark-guided technique." *Saudi J Anaesth*. 2020;14(3):414.
- Er J, Xia J, Gao R, Yu Y. A randomized clinical trial: optimal strategies of paravertebral nerve block combined with general anesthesia for postoperative analgesia in patients undergoing lobectomy: a comparison of the effects of different approaches for serratus anterior plane block. *Ann Palliat Med*. 2021;10(11):11464-11472.
- Lin J, Hoffman T, Badashova K, Motov S, Haines L. Serratus Anterior Plane Block in the Emergency Department: A Case Series. *Clin Pract Cases Emerg Med*. 2020;4(1):21-25.
- Vadera H, Mistry T, Ratre B. Serratus anterior plane block: Anatomical landmark-guided technique. *Saudi J Anaesth*. 2020;14(1):134.
- Xie C, Ran G, Chen D, Lu Y. A narrative review of

ultrasound-guided serratus anterior plane block. *Ann Palliat Med.* 2021;10(1):700-706.

Erector Spinae Plane Block
- Barrios A, Camelo J, Gomez J, et al. Evaluation of Sensory Mapping of Erector Spinae Plane Block. *Pain Physician.* 2020;23(3):E289-E296.
- Chin KJ, El-Boghdadly K. Mechanisms of action of the erector spinae plane (ESP) block: a narrative review. *Can J Anesth/J Can Anesth.* 2021;68(3):387-408.
- Hacibeyoglu G. Arican S, Ulukaya SO, et al. Evaluation of the Efficacy of Erector Spinae Plane Block and Intercostal Nerve Block in the Postherpetic Neuralgia. *Agri.* 2020;32(4):208-218.
- Kot P, Rodriguez P, Granell M, et al. The erector spinae plane block: a narrative review. *Korean J Anesthesiol.* 2019;72(3):209-220.
- White L, Riley B, Malla U, et al. Erector spinae block versus serratus anterior block in chest wall trauma, which is better?: A response and decision making guide. *Am J Emerg Med.* 2020;38(10):2221-2223.

Interscalene Brachial Plexus Block
- Blaivas M, Adhikari S, Lander L. A Prospective Comparison of Procedural Sedation and Ultrasound-guided Interscalene Nerve Block for Shoulder Reduction in the EmergDepartment. *Acad Emerg Med.* 2011;18(9):922-927.
- Gautier P, Vandepitte C, Ramquet C, DeCoopman M, Xu D, Hadzic A. The Minimum Effective Anesthetic Volume of 0.75% Ropivacaine in Ultrasound-Guided Interscalene Brachial Plexus Block. *Anesthesia & Analgesia.* 2011;113(4):951-955.
- Mantuani D, Nagdev A. Sonographic evaluation of a paralyzed hemidiaphragm from ultrasound-guided interscalene brachial plexus nerve block. *Am J Emerg Med.* 2012;30(9):2099.e5-2099.e7.
- Raeyat Doost E, Heiran MM, Movahedi M, Mirafzal A. Ultrasound-guided interscalene nerve block vs procedural sedation by propofol and fentanyl for anterior shoulder dislocations. *Am J Emerg Med.* 2017;35(10):1435-1439.
- Renes SH, Rettig HC, Gielen MJ, Wilder-Smith OH, van Geffen GJ. Ultrasound-Guided Low-Dose Interscalene Brachial Plexus Block Reduces the Incidence of Hemidiaphragmatic Paresis. *Reg Anesth Pain Medicine.* 2009;34(5):498-502.

Supraclavicular Brachial Plexus Block
- Jeon DG, Kim SK, Kang BJ, Kwon MA, Song JG, Jeon SM. Comparison of ultrasound-guided supraclavicular block according to the various volumes of local anesthetic. *Korean J Anesthesiol.* 2013;64(6):494.
- Renes SH, Spoormans HH, Gielen MJ, Rettig HC, van Geffen GJ. Hemidiaphragmatic Paresis Can Be Avoided in Ultrasound-Guided Supraclavicular Brachial Plexus Block. *Reg Anesth Pain Med.* 2009;34(6):595-599.
- Murata H, Sakai A, Hadzic A, Sumikawa K. The Presence of Transverse Cervical and Dorsal Scapular Arteries at Three Ultrasound Probe Positions Commonly Used in Supraclavicular Brachial Plexus Blockade. *Anesthesia & Analgesia.* 2012;115(2):470-473.
- Stone MB, Wang R, Price DD. Ultrasound-guided supraclavicular brachial plexus nerve block vs procedural sedation for the treatment of upper extremity emergencies. *Am J Emerg Med.* 2008;26(6):706-710.

Suprascapular Nerve Block
- Fernandes MR, Barbosa MA, Sousa ALL, Ramos GC. Suprascapular Nerve Block: Important Procedure in Clinical Practice. *Rev Bras Anestesiol.* 2012;62(1):96-104.
- Harmon D, Hearty C. Ultrasound-guided suprascapular nerve block technique. *Pain Physician.* 2007;10(6):743-746.
- Messina C, Banfi G, Orlandi D, et al. Ultrasound-guided interventional procedures around the shoulder. *BJR.* 2016;89(1057):20150372.
- Schoenherr JW, Flynn DN, Doyal A. Suprascapular Nerve Block. In: StatPearls. StatPearls Publishing; 2022. http://www.ncbi.nlm.nih.gov/books/NBK580556/. Accessed July 11, 2022.
- Neal JM, Gerancher JC, Hebl JR, et al. Upper extremity regional anesthesia: essentials of our current understanding, 2008. *Reg Anesth Pain Med.* 2009;34(2):134-170.
- White R, Croft M, Bird S, Sampson M. Ultrasonography-guided common musculoskeletal interventions from head to toe: procedural tips for general radiologists. *Korean J Radiol.* 2021;22(12):2006-2016.

Axillary Brachial Plexus Block
- Bernucci F, Gonzalez AP, Finlayson RJ, Tran DQH. A Prospective, Randomized Comparison Between Perivascular and Perineural Ultrasound-Guided

Axillary Brachial Plexus Block. *Reg Anesth Pain Med.* 2012;37(5):473-477.
- Bigeleisen PE. Nerve Puncture and Apparent Intraneural Injection during Ultrasound-guided Axillary Block Does Not Invariably Result in Neurologic Injury. *Anesthesiology.* 2006;105(4):779-783.
- Chan VWS, Perlas A, McCartney CJL, Brull R, Xu D, Abbas S. Ultrasound guidance improves success rate of axillary brachial plexus block. *Can J Anesth/J Can Anesth.* 2007;54(3):176-182.
- Cho S, Kim YJ, Baik HJ, Kim JH, Woo JH. Comparison of Ultrasound-Guided Axillary Brachial Plexus Block Techniques: Perineural Injection versus Single or Double Perivascular Infiltration. *Yonsei Med J.* 2015;56(3):838.
- Liu FC, Liou JT, Tsai YF, et al. Efficacy of ultrasound-guided axillary brachial plexus block: a comparative study with nerve stimulator-guided method. *Chang Gung Med J.* 2005;28(6):396-402. http://cgmj.cgu.edu.tw/2806/280604.pdf. Accessed June 29, 2022.
- O'Donnell BD, Iohom G. An Estimation of the Minimum Effective Anesthetic Volume of 2% Lidocaine in Ultrasound-guided Axillary Brachial Plexus Block. *Anesthesiology.* 2009;111(1):25-29.
- Ranganath A, Srinivasan KK, Iohom G. Ultrasound guided axillary brachial plexus block. *Med Ultrason.* 2014;16(3).

Ulnar Nerve Block
- Canders CP, Krishna PK, Moheimani RS, Weaver CM. Management of an Acute Exacerbation of Chronic Neuropathic Pain in the Emergency Department: A Case to Support Ultrasound-Guided Forearm Nerve Blocks. *J Emerg Med.* 2018;55(6):e147-e151.
- Choquet O, Capdevila X. Three-Dimensional High-Resolution Ultrasound-Guided Axillary Block: A New Panoramic Vision of Local Anesthetic Spread and Perineural Catheter Tip Location. *Anesthesia & Analgesia.* 2013;116(5):1176-1181.
- Kathirgamanathan A, French J, Foxall GL, Hardman JG, Bedforth NM. Delineation of distal ulnar nerve anatomy using ultrasound in volunteers to identify an optimum approach for neural blockade. *Eur J Anaesthesiol.* 2009;26(1):43-46.
- Li Y, Niu J, Liu T, et al. Conduction Block and Nerve Cross-Sectional Area in Multifocal Motor Neuropathy. *Front Neurol.* 2019;10:1055.
- Liebmann O, Price D, Mills C, et al. Feasibility of Forearm Ultrasonography-Guided Nerve Blocks of the Radial, Ulnar, and Median Nerves for Hand Procedures in the Emergency Department. *Ann Emerg Med.* 2006;48(5):558-562.
- Marhofer D, Kettner SC, Marhofer P, Pils S, Weber M, Zeitlinger M. Dexmedetomidine as an adjuvant to ropivacaine prolongs peripheral nerve block: a volunteer study. *Br J Anaesth.* 2013;110(3):438-442.
- Marhofer P, Columb M, Hopkins PM, et al. Dexamethasone as an adjuvant for peripheral nerve blockade: a randomised, triple-blinded crossover study in volunteers. *Br J Anaesth.* 2019;122(4):525-531.
- Meco BC, Ozcelik M, Oztuna DG, et al. Can we gain an advantage by combining distal median, radial and ulnar nerve blocks with supraclavicular block? A randomized controlled study. *J Anesth.* 2015;29(2):217-222.
- Mori T, Nomura O, Ihara T. Ultrasound-guided peripheral forearm nerve block for digit fractures in a pediatric emergency department. *Am J Emerg Med.* 2019;37(3):489-493.
- Stone MB, Muresanu M. Ultrasound-guided Ulnar Nerve Block in the Management of Digital Abscess and Hand Cellulitis. *Acad Emerg Med.* 2010;17(1):E3-E4.
- Ünlüer EE, Karagöz A, Ünlüer S, Oyar O, Özgürbüz U. Ultrasound-guided ulnar nerve block for boxer fractures. *Am J Emerg Med.* 2016;34(8):1726-1727.
- Vastrad V, Mulimani S, Talikoti D, Sorganvi V. A comparative clinical study of ultrasonography-guided perivascular and perineural axillary brachial plexus block for upper limb surgeries. *Anesth Essays Res.* 2019;13(1):163.

Radial Nerve Block
- Aydin AA, Bilge S, Kaya M, Aydin G, Cinar O. Novel technique in ED: supracondylar ultrasound-guided nerve block for reduction of distal radius fractures. *Am J Emerg Med.* 2016;34(5):912-913.
- Balaban O, Aydın T, Inal S, Yaman M. Ultrasound-guided Mid-humeral Radial Nerve Block Provides Sufficient Surgical Anesthesia at Hand Dorsum: A Novel Method and Report of Three Cases. *Cureus.* 2019;11(1):e3949.
- Bhakta P, Zaheer H. Ultrasound-guided radial nerve block to relieve cannulation-induced radial arterial spasm. *Can J Anesth/J Can Anesth.* 2017;64(12):1269-1270.
- Dufeu N, Marchand-Maillet F, Atchabahian A, et al. Efficacy and Safety of Ultrasound-Guided Distal Blocks for Analgesia Without Motor Blockade After Ambulatory Hand Surgery. *J Hand Surg Am.*

2014;39(4):737-743.
- Ünlüer EE, Karagöz A, Ünlüer S, et al. Ultrasound-guided supracondylar radial nerve block for Colles Fractures in the ED. *Am J Emerg Med.* 2016;34(8):1718-1720.
- Zhu W, Zhou R, Chen L, et al. The ultrasound-guided selective nerve block in the upper arm: an approach of retaining the motor function in elbow. *BMC Anesthesiol.* 2018;18(1):143.

Median Nerve Block
- Frenkel O, Liebmann O, Fischer JW. Ultrasound-guided forearm nerve blocks in kids: a novel method for pain control in the treatment of hand-injured pediatric patients in the emergency department. *Pediatr Emerg Care.* 2015;31(4):255-259.
- Gray AT. Chapter 37: Median Nerve Block. In: Atlas of Ultrasound-Guided Regional Anesthesia. Philadelphia, PA: Elsevier, Inc.; 2019:132-137.
- Liebmann O, Price D, Mills C, et al. Feasibility of forearm ultrasonography-guided nerve blocks of the radial, ulnar, and median nerves for hand procedures in the emergency department. *Ann Emerg Med.* 2006;48(5):558-562.
- Sehmbi H, Madjdpour C, Shah UJ, Chin KJ. Ultrasound guided distal peripheral nerve block of the upper limb: A technical review. *J Anaesthesiol Clin Pharmacol.* 2015;31(3):296-307.
- Vrablik M, Akhavan A, Murphy D, Schrepel C, Hall MK. Ultrasound-Guided Nerve Blocks for Painful Hand Injuries: A Randomized Control Trial. *Cureus.* 2021;13(10):e18978. Published 2021 Oct 22. doi:10.7759/cureus.18978
- Yurgil JL, Hulsopple CD, Leggit JC. Nerve Blocks: Part I. Upper Extremity. *Am Fam Physician.* 2020;101(11):654-664.

Landmark Based Hand Block
- Ferreres A, Foucher G, Suso S. Extensive denervation of the wrist. *Tech Hand Up Extrem Surg.* 2002;6(1):36-41.
- Kocheta A, Agrawal Y. Landmark Technique for a Wrist Block. *JBJS Essent Surg Tech.* 2018;8(1):e7. Published 2018 Mar 14.
- Prithishkumar IJ, Joy P, Satyanandan C. Comparison of the volar and medial approach in peripheral block of ulnar nerve at the wrist – a cadaveric study. *J Clin Diagn Res.* 2014;8(1):AC01-AC4.
- Sohoni A, Nagdev A, Takhar S, Stone M. Forearm ultrasound-guided nerve blocks vs landmark-based wrist blocks for hand anesthesia in healthy volunteers. *Am J Emerg Med.* 2016;34(4):730-734.
- Yurgil JL, Hulsopple CD, Leggit JC. Nerve Blocks: Part I. Upper Extremity. *Am Fam Physician.* 2020;101(11):654-664.

PENG Block
- Acharya U, Lamsal R. Pericapsular Nerve Group Block: An Excellent Option for Analgesia for Positional Pain in Hip Fractures. *Case Rep Anesth.* 2020;2020:1-3.
- Berlioz BE, Bojaxhi E. PENG Regional Block. In: StatPearls. StatPearls Publishing; 2022. http://www.ncbi.nlm.nih.gov/books/NBK565870/. Accessed June 29, 2022.
- Kukreja P, Avila A, Northern T, Dangle J, Kolli S, Kalagara H. A Retrospective Case Series of Pericapsular Nerve Group (PENG) Block for Primary Versus Revision Total Hip Arthroplasty Analgesia. *Cureus.* Online May 19, 2020.
- Lin DY, Morrison C, Brown B, et al. Pericapsular nerve group (PENG) block provides improved short-term analgesia compared with the femoral nerve block in hip fracture surgery: a single-center double-blinded randomized comparative trial. *Reg Anesth Pain Med.* 2021;46(5):398-403.
- Rocha-Romero A, Arias-Mejia K, Salas-Ruiz A, Peng PWH. Pericapsular nerve group (PENG) block for hip fracture in the emergency department: a case series. *Anaesthesia Reports.* 2021;9(1):97-100.

Transgluteal Sciatic Nerve Block
- Alsatli R. Comparison of ultrasound-guided anterior versus transgluteal sciatic nerve blockade for knee surgery. *Anesth Essays Res.* 2012;6(1):29.
- Goldsmith AJ, Liteplo A, Hayes BD, Duggan N, Huang C, Shokoohi H. Ultrasound-guided transgluteal sciatic nerve analgesia for refractory back pain in the ED. *Am J Emerg Med.* 2020;38(9):1792-1795.
- Nwawka OK, Meyer R, Miller TT. Ultrasound-Guided Subgluteal Sciatic Nerve Perineural Injection: Report on Safety and Efficacy at a Single Institution. *J Ultrasound Med.* 2017;36(11):2319-2324.
- Selame LA, McFadden K, Duggan NM, Goldsmith AJ, Shokoohi H. Ultrasound-Guided Transgluteal Sciatic Nerve Block for Gluteal Procedural Analgesia. *J Emerg Med.* 2021;60(4):512-516.
- van Geffen GJ, Pirotte T, Gielen MJ, Scheffer G, Bruhn J. Ultrasound-guided proximal and distal sciatic nerve blocks in children. *J Clin Anesth.*

- Yamamoto H, Sakura S, Wada M, Shido A. A Prospective, Randomized Comparison Between Single- and Multiple-Injection Techniques for Ultrasound-Guided Subgluteal Sciatic Nerve Block. *Anesthesia & Analgesia.* 2014;119(6):1442-1448.
- Yoshida T, Nakamoto T, Hashimoto C, Aihara S, Nishimoto K, Kamibayashi T. An Ultrasound-Guided Lateral Approach for Proximal Sciatic Nerve Block: A Randomized Comparison With the Anterior Approach and a Cadaveric Evaluation. *Reg Anesth Pain Med.* Published online July 2018:1.

Fascia Iliaca Block

- Beaudoin FL, Haran JP, Liebmann O. A Comparison of Ultrasound-guided Three-in-one Femoral Nerve Block Versus Parenteral Opioids Alone for Analgesia in Emergency Department Patients With Hip Fractures: A Randomized Controlled Trial. Miner JR, ed. *Acad Emerg Med.* 2013;20(6):584-591.
- Cooper AL, Nagree Y, Goudie A, Watson PR, Arendts G. Ultrasound-guided femoral nerve blocks are not superior to ultrasound-guided fascia iliaca blocks for fractured neck of femur. *Emerg Med Australas.* 2019;31(3):393-398.
- Dickman E, Pushkar I, Likourezos A, et al. Ultrasound-guided nerve blocks for intracapsular and extracapsular hip fractures. *Am J Emerg Med.* 2016;34(3):586-589.
- Ketelaars R, Stollman JT, van Eeten E, Eikendal T, Bruhn J, van Geffen GJ. Emergency physician-performed ultrasound-guided nerve blocks in proximal femoral fractures provide safe and effective pain relief: a prospective observational study in The Netherlands. *Int J Emerg Med.* 2018;11(1):12.
- Morrison RS, Dickman E, Hwang U, et al. Regional Nerve Blocks Improve Pain and Functional Outcomes in Hip Fracture: A Randomized Controlled Trial. *J Am Geriatr Soc.* 2016;64(12):2433-2439.
- Topal FE, Bilgin S, Yamanoglu A, et al. The Feasibility of the Ultrasound-Guided Femoral Nerve Block Procedure with Low-Dose Local Anesthetic in Intracapsular and Extracapsular Hip Fractures. *J Emerg Med.* 2020;58(4):553–561.

Saphenous Nerve / Adductor Canal Block

- Burckett-St. Laurant D, Peng P, Girón Arango L, et al. The Nerves of the Adductor Canal and the Innervation of the Knee: An Anatomic Study. *Reg Anesth Pain Med.* 2016;41(3):321-327.
- Davis JJ, Bond TS, Swenson JD. Adductor Canal Block: More Than Just the Saphenous Nerve? *Reg Anesth Pain Med.* 2009;34(6):618-619.
- Eglitis N, Horn JL, Benninger B, Nelsen S. The Importance of the Saphenous Nerve in Ankle Surgery. *Anesthesia & Analgesia.* 2016;122(5):1704-1706.
- Fei Y, Cui X, Chen S, et al. Continuous block at the proximal end of the adductor canal provides better analgesia compared to that at the middle of the canal after total knee arthroplasty: a randomized, double-blind, controlled trial. *BMC Anesthesiol.* 2020;20(1):260.
- Gadsden J, Warlick A. Regional anesthesia for the trauma patient: improving patient outcomes. *Local Reg Anesth.* 2015;8:45-55.
- Kendir S, Torun BI, Akkaya T, Comert A, Tuccar E, Tekdemir I. Re-defining the anatomical structures for blocking the nerves in adductor canal and sciatic nerve through the same injection site: an anatomical study. *Surg Radiol Anat.* 2018;40(11):1267-1274.
- Marsland D, Dray A, Little NJ, Solan MC. The saphenous nerve in foot and ankle surgery: Its variable anatomy and relevance. *Foot Ankle Surg.* 2013;19(2):76-79.
- Panchamia JK, Niesen AD, Amundson AW. Adductor Canal Versus Femoral Triangle: Let Us All Get on the Same Page. *Anesthesia & Analgesia.* 2018;127(3):e50.
- Pascarella G, Costa F, Del Buono R, Agrò F. Adductor canal and femoral triangle: Two different rooms with the same door. *Saudi J Anaesth.* 2019;13(3):276.
- Ranganath YS, Yap A, Wong CA, Ravindranath S, Marian AA. Adductor Canal Blocks: An Observational Ultrasound Study in Volunteers to Identify the Relationship of the True Adductor Canal to Commonly Described Block Approaches and a Review of the Literature. In Review; 2019. DOI:10.21203/rs.2.11977/v1.
- Sondekoppam RV, Johnston DF, Ranganath YS, Parra MC, Marian AA. Adductor canal or femoral triangle block: the continuity conundrum. *Br J Anaesth.* 2020;124(4):e194-e195.
- Song L, Li Y, Xu Z, Geng ZY, Wang DX. Comparison of the ultrasound-guided single-injection femoral triangle block versus adductor canal block for analgesia following total knee arthroplasty: a randomized, double-blind trial. *J Anesth.*

2020;34(5):702-711.
- Wong WY, Bjørn S, Strid JMC, Børglum J, Bendtsen TF. Defining the Location of the Adductor Canal Using Ultrasound. *Reg Anesth Pain Med*. 2017;42(2):241-245.

Distal Sciatic Nerve Block in the Popliteal Fossa
- Bang SU, Kim DJ, Bae JH, Chung K, Kim Y. Minimum effective local anesthetic volume for surgical anesthesia by subparaneural, ultrasound-guided popliteal sciatic nerve block: A prospective dose-finding study. *Medicine (Baltimore)*. 2016;95(34):e4652.
- Barbosa FT, Barbosa TRBW, da Cunha RM, Rodrigues AKB, da Silva Ramos FW, de Sousa-Rodrigues CF. Anatomical basis for sciatic nerve block at the knee level. *Braz J Anesthesiol*. 2015;65(3):177-179.
- Cappelleri G, Ambrosoli AL, Gemma M, Cedrati VLE, Bizzarri F, Danelli GF. Intraneural Ultrasound-guided Sciatic Nerve Block. *Anesthesiology*. 2018;129(2):241-248.
- David S, Varghese D, Valiaveedan S. What is the minimum effective anesthetic volume (MEAV90) of 0.2% ropivacaine required for ultrasound-guided popliteal-sciatic nerve block? *J Anaesthesiol Clin Pharmacol*. 2021;37(3):402.
- Wiederhold BD, Garmon EH, Peterson E, Stevens JB, O'Rourke MC. Nerve Block Anesthesia. In: StatPearls. StatPearls Publishing; 2022. http://www.ncbi.nlm.nih.gov/books/NBK431109/. Accessed July 11, 2022

Ankle Block
- Allam AE, Mansour ER. Superficial Peroneal Nerve Block. In: StatPearls. Treasure Island (FL): StatPearls Publishing; September 5, 2022.
- Arnold C, Alvarado AC, Brady MF. Saphenous Nerve Block. In: StatPearls. Treasure Island (FL): StatPearls Publishing; May 29, 2022.
- Chan T, Wilkinson A, Hendrick S. A Technique Guide in Ultrasound Guided Regional Ankle Blocks. *J Foot Ankle Surg*. 2021;60(4):817-823.
- Chin KJ, Wong NW, Macfarlane AJ, Chan VW. Ultrasound-guided versus anatomic landmark-guided ankle blocks: a 6-year retrospective review. *Reg Anesth Pain Med*. 2011;36(6):611-618.
- Davies T, Karanovic S, Shergill B. Essential regional nerve blocks for the dermatologist: Part 2. *Clin Exp Dermatol*. 2014;39(8):861-867.
- Delbos A, Philippe M, Clément C, Olivier R, Coppens S. Ultrasound-guided ankle block. History revisited. *Best Pract Res Clin Anaesthesiol*. 2019;33(1):79-93.
- Gray AT. Chapter 48: Ankle Blocks. In: Atlas of Ultrasound-Guided Regional Anesthesia. Philadelphia, PA: Elsevier, Inc.; 2019:204-204.
- Yurgil JL, Hulsopple CD, Leggit JC. Nerve Blocks: Part II. Lower Extremity. *Am Fam Physician*. 2020;101(11):669-679.

Distal Tibial Nerve Block
- Chin KJ, Wong NWY, Macfarlane AJR, Chan VWS. Ultrasound-Guided Versus Anatomic Landmark-Guided Ankle Blocks: A 6-Year Retrospective Review. Reg Anesth Pain Med. 2011;36(6):611-618.
- Clattenburg E, Herring A, Hahn C, Johnson B, Nagdev A. ED ultrasound-guided posterior tibial nerve blocks for calcaneal fracture analgesia. *Am J Emerg Med*. 2016;34(6):1183.e1-1183.e3.
- Moake MM, Presley BC, Barnes RM. Ultrasound-Guided Posterior Tibial Nerve Block for Plantar Foot Foreign Body Removal. *Pediatr Emerg Care*. 2020;36(5):262-265.
- Redborg KE, Antonakakis JG, Beach ML, Chinn CD, Sites BD. Ultrasound Improves the Success Rate of a Tibial Nerve Block at the Ankle. *Reg Anesth Pain Med*. 2009;34(3):256-260.
- Soares LG, Brull R, Chan VW. Teaching an old block a new trick: ultrasound-guided posterior tibial nerve block: Letters to the Editor. *Acta Anaesthesiologica Scandinavica*. 2008;52(3):446-447.

Hematoma Block for Humerus Fractures
- Ross A, Catanzariti AR, Mendicino RW. The Hematoma Block: A Simple, Effective Technique for Closed Reduction of Ankle Fracture Dislocations. *J Foot Ankle Surg*. 2011;50(4):507-509.
- Urfalioglu A, Gokdemir O, Hanbeyoglu O, et al. A comparison of ankle block and spinal anesthesia for foot surgery. 2015;8(10):19388-19393. https://www.ncbi.nlm.nih.gov/pmc/articles/PMC4694480/. Accessed July 11, 2022

Hematoma Block for Ankle Fractures
- Gottlieb M, Cosby K. Ultrasound-guided Hematoma Block for Distal Radial and Ulnar Fractures. *J Emerg Med*. 2015;48(3):310-312.
- Maleitzke T, Plachel F, Fleckenstein FN, Wichlas F, Tsitsilonis S. Haematoma block: a safe method for pre-surgical reduction of distal radius fractures. *J Orthop Surg Res*. 2020;15(1):351.
- Orbach H, Rozen N, Rinat B, Rubin G. Hematoma block for distal radius fractures – prospective, randomized comparison of two different volumes

of lidocaine. *J Int Med Res.* 2018;46(11):4535-4538.
- Tseng PT, Leu TH, Chen YW, Chen YP. Hematoma block or procedural sedation and analgesia, which is the most effective method of anesthesia in reduction of displaced distal radius fracture? *J Orthop Surg Res.* 2018;13(1):62.

Hematoma Block for Wrist Fractures
- Bear DM, Friel NA, Lupo CL, Pitetti R, Ward WT. Hematoma Block Versus Sedation for the Reduction of Distal Radius Fractures in Children. *J Hand Surg Am.* 2015;40(1):57-61.
- Fathi M, Moezzi M, Abbasi S, Farsi D, Zare MA, Hafezimoghadam P. Ultrasound-guided hematoma block in distal radial fracture reduction: a randomised clinical trial. *Emerg Med J.* 2015;32(6):474-477.
- Gottlieb M, Cosby K. Ultrasound-guided Hematoma Block for Distal Radial and Ulnar Fractures. *J Emerg Med.* 2015;48(3):310-312.
- Maleitzke T, Plachel F, Fleckenstein FN, Wichlas F, Tsitsilonis S. Haematoma block: a safe method for pre-surgical reduction of distal radius fractures. *J Orthop Res.* 2020;15(1):351.
- Siebelt M, Hartholt KA, van Winden DFM, et al. Ultrasound-Guided Nerve Blocks as Analgesia for Nonoperative Management of Distal Radius Fractures—Two Consecutive Randomized Controlled Trials. *J Orthop Trauma.* 2019;33(4):e124-e130.
- Tseng PT, Leu TH, Chen YW, Chen YP. Hematoma block or procedural sedation and analgesia, which is the most effective method of anesthesia in reduction of displaced distal radius fracture? *J Orthop Surg Res.* 2018;13(1):62.

TPI Thoracic and Lumbar Muscles
- Alvarez DJ, Rockwell PG. Trigger points: diagnosis and management. *Am Fam Physician.* 2002;65(4):653-660. https://www.aafp.org/pubs/afp/issues/2002/0215/p653.html. Accessed June 29, 2022.
- Botwin KP, Sharma K, Saliba R, Patel BC. Ultrasound-guided trigger point injections in the cervicothoracic musculature: a new and unreported technique. *Pain Physician.* 2008;11(6):885-889. Accessed June 29, 2022.
- Garvey TA, Marks MR, Wiesel SW. A Prospective, Randomized, Double-Blind Evaluation of Trigger-Point Injection Therapy for Low-Back Pain. *Spine.* 1989;14(9):962-964.
- Hammi C, Schroeder JD, Yeung B. Trigger Point Injection. In: StatPearls. StatPearls Publishing; 2022. http://www.ncbi.nlm.nih.gov/books/NBK542196/. Accessed July 6, 2022.
- Lavelle ED, Lavelle W, Smith HS. Myofascial Trigger Points. *Med Clin North Am.* 2007;91(2):229-239.
- Sikdar S, Shah JP, Gebreab T, et al. Novel Applications of Ultrasound Technology to Visualize and Characterize Myofascial Trigger Points and Surrounding Soft Tissue. *Arch Phys Med Rehabil.* 2009;90(11):1829-1838.
- Wong CSM, Wong SHS. A New Look at Trigger Point Injections. *Anesthesiol Res Pract.* 2012;2012:1-5.

TPI Cervical and Trapezius Muscles
- Alvarez DJ, Rockwell PG. Trigger points: diagnosis and management. *Am Fam Physician.* 2002;65(4):653-660. Accessed June 29, 2022.
- Botwin KP, Sharma K, Saliba R, Patel BC. Ultrasound-guided trigger point injections in the cervicothoracic musculature: a new and unreported technique. *Pain Physician.* 2008;11(6):885-889. Accessed June 29, 2022.
- Garvey TA, Marks MR, Wiesel SW. A Prospective, Randomized, Double-Blind Evaluation of Trigger-Point Injection Therapy for Low-Back Pain. *Spine.* 1989;14(9):962-964.
- Hammi C, Schroeder JD, Yeung B. Trigger Point Injection. In: StatPearls. StatPearls Publishing; 2022. http://www.ncbi.nlm.nih.gov/books/NBK542196/. Accessed June 29, 2022.
- Lavelle ED, Lavelle W, Smith HS. Myofascial Trigger Points. *Med Clin North Am.* 2007;91(2):229-239.
- Sikdar S, Shah JP, Gebreab T, et al. Novel Applications of Ultrasound Technology to Visualize and Characterize Myofascial Trigger Points and Surrounding Soft Tissue. *Arch Phys Med Rehabil.* 2009;90(11):1829-1838.
- Tsai CT, Hsieh LF, Kuan TS, Kao MJ, Chou LW, Hong CZ. Remote Effects of Dry Needling on the Irritability of the Myofascial Trigger Point in the Upper Trapezius Muscle. *Am J Phys Med Rehabil.* 2010;89(2):133-140.
- Wong CSM, Wong SHS. A New Look at Trigger Point Injections. *Anesthesiol Res Pract.* 2012;2012:1-5.

Knee Injections
- Adhikari S, Blaivas M. Utility of bedside sonography to distinguish soft tissue abnormalities from joint effusions in the emergency department. *J Ultrasound Med.* 2010;29(4):519-526.

- Berkoff DJ, Miller LE, Block JE. Clinical utility of ultrasound guidance for intra-articular knee injections: a review. *Clin Interv Aging*. 2012;7:89-95.
- Johnson B, Lovallo E, Mantuani D, Nagdev A. How to perform ultrasound-guided knee arthrocentesis. ACEP Now. Published August 13, 2015. Accessed February 21, 2023.
- Roberts JR, Custalow CB, Thomsen TW. Chapter 53: Arthrocentesis. In: Roberts and Hedges' Clinical Procedures in Emergency Medicine and Acute Care. Philadelphia, PA: Elsevier; 2019.
- Sibbitt WL Jr, Kettwich LG, Band PA, et al. Does ultrasound guidance improve the outcomes of arthrocentesis and corticosteroid injection of the knee?. *Scand J Rheumatol*. 2012;41(1):66-72.
- Tieng A, Franchin G. Knee Arthrocentesis in Adults. *J Vis Exp*. 2022;(180):10.3791/63135. Published 2022 Feb 25.
- Wiler JL, Costantino TG, Filippone L, Satz W. Comparison of ultrasound-guided and standard landmark techniques for knee arthrocentesis. *J Emerg Med*. 2010;39(1):76-82.

Shoulder Injections
- Aly AR, Rajasekaran S, Ashworth N. Ultrasound-guided shoulder girdle injections are more accurate and more effective than landmark-guided injections: a systematic review and meta-analysis. *Br J Sports Med*. 2015;49(16):1042-1049.
- Kuratani K, Tanaka M, Hanai H, Hayashida K. Accuracy of shoulder joint injections with ultrasound guidance: Confirmed by magnetic resonance arthrography. *World J Orthop*. 2022;13(3):259-266. Published 2022 Mar 18.
- Miller SL, Cleeman E, Auerbach J, Flatow EL. Comparison of intra-articular lidocaine and intravenous sedation for reduction of shoulder dislocations: a randomized, prospective study. *J Bone Joint Surg Am*. 2002;84(12):2135-2139.
- Nagdev A. Ultrasound-Guided Glenohumeral Joint Evaluation and Aspiration. ACEP Now. Published June 15, 2016. Accessed February 21, 2023.
- Patel DN, Nayyar S, Hasan S, Khatib O, Sidash S, Jazrawi LM. Comparison of ultrasound-guided versus blind glenohumeral injections: a cadaveric study. *J Shoulder Elbow Surg*. 2012;21(12):1664-1668.
- Waterbrook AL, Paul S. Intra-articular Lidocaine Injection for Shoulder Reductions: A Clinical Review. *Sports Health*. 2011;3(6):556-559.

Hip Injections
- Anderson ES, Herring AA, Bailey C, Mantuani D, Nagdev AD. Ultrasound-guided Intraarticular Hip Injection for Osteoarthritisv in the Emergency Department. *West J Emerg Med*. 2013;14(5):505-508.
- Bailey C, Mantuani D, Nagdev A. Bedside Ultrasound for the Septic Hip. ACEP Now. Published June 1, 2012. Accessed February 21, 2023.
- Boniface K, Pyle M, Jaleesah N, Shokoohi H. Point-of-Care Ultrasound for the Detection of Hip Effusion and Septic Arthritis in Adult Patients With Hip Pain and Negative Initial Imaging. *J Emerg Med*. 2020;58(4):627-631.
- Freeman K, Dewitz A, Baker WE. Ultrasound-guided hip arthrocentesis in the ED. *Am J Emerg Med*. 2007;25(1):80-86.
- Ma OJ, Mateer JR, Reardon RF, Joing S. Ma and Mateer's Emergency Ultrasound. 3rd ed. New York, NY: McGraw-Hill Education; 2014.

Evidence of Benefit
- Amini R, Kartchner JZ, Nagdev A, Adhikari S. Ultrasound-Guided Nerve Blocks in Emergency Medicine Practice. *J Ultrasound Med*. 2016;35(4):731-736.
- Gadsden J, Warlick A. Regional anesthesia for the trauma patient: improving patient outcomes. Local *Reg Anesth*. 2015;8:45-55. Published 2015 Aug 12.
- Malik A, Thom S, Haber B, et al. Regional Anesthesia in the Emergency Department: an Overview of Common Nerve Block Techniques and Recent Literature. *Curr Emerg Hosp Med Rep*. 2022;10:54–66.
- Tucker RV, Peterson WJ, Mink JT, et al. Defining an Ultrasound-guided Regional Anesthesia Curriculum for Emergency Medicine. *AEM Educ Train*. 2020;5(3):e10557.
- Walker KJ, McGrattan K, Aas-Eng K, Smith AF. Ultrasound guidance for peripheral nerve blockade. *Cochrane Database Syst Rev*. 2009;(4):CD006459.

How to Implement Regional Anesthesia Training
- Amini R, Kartchner JZ, Nagdev A, Adhikari S. Ultrasound-Guided Nerve Blocks in Emergency Medicine Practice. J Ultrasound Med Off J Am Inst Ultrasound Med. 2016;35(4):731-736.
- Herring AA. Bringing Ultrasound-guided Regional Anesthesia to Emergency Medicine. *AEM Educ Train*. 2017;1(2):165-168.

- Johnson B, Herring A, Shah S, Krosin M, Mantuani D, Nagdev A. Door-to-block time: prioritizing acute pain management for femoral fractures in the ED. *Am J Emerg Med*. 2014;32(7):801-803.
- Levene JL, Weinstein EJ, Cohen MS, et al. Local anesthetics and regional anesthesia versus conventional analgesia for preventing persistent postoperative pain in adults and children: A Cochrane systematic review and meta-analysis update. *J Clin Anesth*. 2019;55:116-127.
- Lin DY, Woodman R, Oberai T, et al. Association of anesthesia and analgesia with long-term mortality after hip fracture surgery: an analysis of the Australian and New Zealand hip fracture registry. *Reg Anesth Pain Med*. 2023;48(1):14-21.
- Morrison RS, Dickman E, Hwang U, et al. Regional Nerve Blocks Improve Pain and Functional Outcomes in Hip Fracture: A Randomized Controlled Trial. *J Am Geriatr Soc*. 2016;64(12):2433-2439.
- Gibson RN, Gibson KI. A home-made phantom for learning ultrasound-guided invasive techniques. *Australas Radiol*. 1995;39(4):356-357.
- Nagdev A, Howell K, Desai A, Martin D, Mantuani D. How To Build an Ultrasound-Guided Nerve Block Program. *ACEP Now*. https://www.acepnow.com/article/how-to-build-an-ultrasound-guided-nerve-block-program/?singlepage=1. Published January 6, 2023. Accessed February 21, 2023.
- Schultz C, Yang E, Mantuani D, Miraflor E, Victorino G, Nagdev A. Single injection, ultrasound-guided planar nerve blocks: An essential skill for any clinician caring for patients with rib fractures. *Trauma Case Rep*. 2022;41:100680.
- Ultrasound Guidelines: Emergency, Point-of-Care and Clinical Ultrasound Guidelines in Medicine. *Ann Emerg Med*. 2017;69(5):e27-e54.
- Wroe P, O'Shea R, Johnson B, Hoffman R, Nagdev A. Ultrasound-guided forearm nerve blocks for hand blast injuries: case series and multidisciplinary protocol. *Am J Emerg Med*. 2016;34(9):1895-1897.

Reimbursement
- Centers for Medicare & Medicaid Services. Medicare Physician Fee Schedule Final Rule Summary: CY 2023. MLN Matters. MM12982. Implementation date Jan. 3, 2023.

INDEX

A

Adductor canal 66
Ankle block 70
Ankle fracture, hematoma block 77
Axillary brachial plexus 46

B

Benefits of RA 9, 92
Block box 93
Brachial plexus
 - Axillary 46
 - Interscalene 40
 - Supraclavicular 42

C

Cervical/trapezius muscle TPI 82
Classes of anesthetics 9, 10
CPT Codes for RA 98
Credentialing 96

D

Distal sciatic nerve in popliteal fossa ..68
Distal tibial nerve 72
Documentation 94
Dosing considerations 11

E

Education 95
Erector spinae plane 34

F

Fascia iliaca 64
Femoral nerve block......................65

G

Greater auricular nerve block 18

H

Hand block, landmark-based 54
Hematoma blocks
 - Humerus fractures 76
 - Ankle fractures 77
 - Wrist fractures 78
Hip injection 88
Humerus fracture, hematoma block 76

I

Infraorbital nerve block 24
Interscalene brachial plexus 40
Infrainguinal fascia iliaco block......64

J

Joint injection
 - Ankle 70, 77
 - Hip 88
 - Shoulder 86
 - Wrist 78

K

Knee injection 84

L

Landmark-based hand block 54
LAST ....13, 14, Back cover
Lidocaine toxicity 14
Lower extremity nerves 59
Lumbar/thoracic muscle TPI 80

M

Max dosage chart 10
Median nerve 52, 56
Mental nerve block 26

N

Needle selection 13
Nerve injury 12

O

Occipital nerve block 20

P

Pectoralis I and II 30
PENG block (periscapular nerve group) . 60
Popliteal fossa 68

R

Radial nerve 50, 57
References 100
Regional analgesia training 93
Reimbursement 97
Reimbursement charts 98
Risks 11

S

Safety protocols 12
Saphenous nerve/adductor canal 66
Sciatic nerve
 - Transgluteal 62
 - Distal 68
Serratus anterior plane 32
Shoulder injection 86
Superficial cervical plexus block 16
Supraclavicular brachial plexus 42
Supraorbital nerve block 22
Suprascapular 44

T

TAP block 36
Thoracic/lumbar muscle TPI 80
Tibial nerve, distal 72
Transgluteal sciatic nerve 62
Transverse Abdominus Plane 36
Trapezius/cervical muscle TPI 82
Trigger point injection
 - Thoracic and lumbar muscles 80
 - Cervical & trapezius muscles .... 82"
Trunk and torso 29

U

Ulnar nerve 48, 56
Ultrasound-guided regional anesthesia
9, 10, 93

W

Wrist fracture, hematoma block 78

Z

Zygomaticofacial nerve 15
Zygomaticotemporal nerve 15